It Started in a Cupboard

Adventures in Life, Learning and Happiness

By the Same Author:

Basic Skills for Surgical Housemen (Churchill Livingstone, 1971)
An Introduction to Surgical Aspects of Haemodialysis (Churchill Livingstone, 1974)
with PRF Bell *Cancer Medicine* (Palgrave Macmillan, 1978) with J Paul
Basic Principles of Cancer Chemotherapy (Palgrave Macmillan, 1980) with MHN
Tattersall and J F Smyth
Basic Skills in Clinical Medicine (Churchill Livingstone, 1984) with C Hanning
Invasion: Experimental and Clinical Implications (Oxford University Press, 1984)
with M Mareel
Nutritional Support for the Cancer Patient (Saunders, 1986) with K Fearon
Living with Cancer: An Introduction for Patients, Families and Staff (Tak Tent, 1987,
privately published) with M Duthie
Royal Medico-Chirurgical Society of Glasgow: A History (1989) with DA Dow
Healthy Respect: Ethics in Health Care (Faber, 1994) with RS Downie
The Potential for Health (Oxford University Press, 1998)
Risk Communication and the Public Health (Oxford University Press, 1999) Edited
with P Bennett
Storytelling, Humour and Learning in Medicine (The Stationery Office, London, 2001)
Oxford Textbook of Palliative Medicine (Oxford University Press, 2005) Joint Editor
with Derek Doyle, Geoffrey Hanks and Nathan Cherny
Handing on Learning: Medical Education: Past present and future (Elsevier 2007)
A Doctor's Line: Poetry and Prescriptions in Health and Healing (Sandstone Press, 2014)
Afterthoughts (Kennedy and Boyd, 2017)

It Started in a Cupboard
Adventures in Life, Learning and Happiness

KENNETH CALMAN

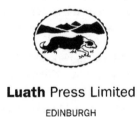

Luath Press Limited

EDINBURGH

www.luath.co.uk

First published 2019

ISBN: 978-1912147-58-8

Printed and bound by
CPI Antony Rowe, Chippenham

Typeset in 11.5 point Sabon by Main Point Books, Edinburgh

Contents

This book is dedicated to my wife Ann, my three children Andrew, Lynn and Susan and their partners, who have helped and supported me over the years and have given me fun, laughter and love, and to my two grandchildren, Grace and Brodie.

Foreword

Compiled by Susan Calman

ALL THREE OF us Calman children breathed a sigh of relief when Dad told us that he was finally writing the story of his life. For a man who is so well known, there are many things that we have never talked about. To have his memories preserved in the pages of this book means that we can fully appreciate his life and achievements, and my niece and nephew will understand that their Grumps (that's their nickname for him, not a comment on his temperament) isn't just a fun-filled man who wears Christmas jumpers; he's a pioneer and a great man.

Rather than me trying to summarise what we all felt, I asked my brother Andrew and sister Lynn to read the book and then send me their thoughts. They echo my own in many ways.

Andrew noted:

There aren't too many people who have done quite as much with their life as Dad has with his, yet when I think of him, I don't think of his achievements so much as the times we've spent together walking the dogs, relaxed in each other's company and putting the world to rights. Even today, those walks mean everything to me

Reading this book made me realise just how much Dad was doing in his professional life while chatting with me about mine. The book is full of references to people, places and events that I remember but did not fully understand at the time, such as Tak Tent meetings at our house, colleagues and friends of his we would bump into, no matter where we were in the world, or seeing him in the news discussing something related to his jobs such as being Chief Medical Officer.

This book has brought back a whole heap of memories of all the places we have lived in, of all the dogs we've had over the years and all the various places we have walked them. Significantly, this book connects memories of different stages of my life through each of these dogs depending on where we were and what we were doing at the time. From being a toddler on Wimbledon Common chasing after Bart, our black Labrador – the first of our family's dogs – to ambling ahead of Ailsa, his slow, snuffling beagle, those walks with Dad have helped shape my past, present and future life, and I treasure them

To this day we all get together on 2 January every year, no matter what else is happening in the world, for a long walk with the dogs. And for all of us it is a chance to connect and relax.

My sister Lynn is the only one of us who has carried on the family tradition of health care. Personally, I faint at the sight of blood so would have been worse than useless in a ward, but she understands Dad's legacy in a different way.

She says:

There can be few people who have had such an impact on the lives of people living with cancer, both at an individual and service delivery level.

I remember as a child visiting his unit at the hospital in Glasgow every Christmas Day – not realising till much later the impact this had on me. But leading the team by example and being there on the ward was so important to him. Despite his regular absences – evenings and Saturday mornings back in the hospital, conferences and courses all over the world – I think we somehow understood even as young children that what he did was so important for people. The smell of a hospital still reminds me of hugging him when he came home at night

He went above and beyond to be there for patients. The team in his unit was truly multidisciplinary with value placed on the role of everyone. The ground-breaking patient booklets written with patients and nurses are an example of this and were well ahead of the curve of what would now be the standard of care in the NHS. I remember hearing the unit 'parties' and skits from my bedroom and thinking whatever they do at work it must be great fun! Back then, I wouldn't have had any inkling of the strain that poor survival rates and limited treatment options would have placed on the team.

Dad's influence in cancer care has gone beyond the individual. The 1995 Calman-Hine report was the first comprehensive report on cancer in the UK and set out a radical change in service delivery for cancer patients, a model that is still used today. This has had an impact on millions of people with cancer; its importance cannot be overstated. He believes he is no longer relevant in the area but his impact can still be seen in oncology practice today.

Dad has been an inspiration in what I do and how I do it. I have followed his path to some extent, although I couldn't match his professorship at 32! I became a nurse and now lead a programme of research in living with and beyond cancer – essentially what the patient-focused care and psycho-oncology, pioneered in his unit, has become – and I am so proud when his contributions are still mentioned at oncology meetings and conferences.

I can't talk about Dad without mentioning Mum, in her own right a role model. She undertook health promotion research with primary school children in the 1980s that was ahead of its time and latterly chaired a large primary care trust in the north-east of England. Without her support and understanding none of the above would have been possible!

I also remember Christmas Days spent visiting the Oncology Ward in Glasgow. And the memories of those times mean that I still have a deep connection to his work. I'm a patron of the charity that Dad set up, Cancer Support Scotland, and also of Target Ovarian Cancer. I can't carry on the research work that he and my sister have been part of, but I can help in a small way to carry on the family legacy.

For me, it is the first few chapters of the book that are the most important. I'm named after my gran, Grace, and she looked after me in the house in Knightswood (described in loving detail in this book) while Mum was at work. So much of hers and my dad's lives were never talked about because it was extremely painful to discuss. The grief over the loss of his father and the struggles that Gran had bringing up two boys on her own are brought vividly to the fore in these pages. It was a revelation to me to finally read the stories and imagine the hardships that the whole family went through. This book has allowed me to know my wonderful gran more as well and that is a priceless, accidental memento.

It's difficult to find a way to conclude a Foreword to a book, as you probably haven't read it yet and I'd hate to spoil the journey for you. What I will say is this. Everyone always says that I'm the spitting image of my father and that's always been a great compliment. After reading the story of his life – and I'm sure I speak for my brother and sister – we are all even more proud to call him our dad.

Andrew, Lynn and Susan Calman
July 2019

CHAPTER I

A Cupboard in Knightswood

I WAS BORN on a day of peace in a world at war. At seven o'clock in the evening on Thursday 25 December 1941, when I came into the world, the BBC's Home Service was about to broadcast the Christmas Night Troop Service from the Church of the Holy Trinity in Bethlehem. On the other side of the world, on that very day, one of my cousins was killed when the Japanese occupied Hong Kong.

In the Lindores Nursing Home, in the West End of Glasgow, none of that registered. There was no radio in the delivery room, and in any case the news of the fall of Hong Kong had been deliberately held back. To Arthur and Grace Calman, the wider world faded into the background. All that mattered was that their first child had been born, weighed a healthy 7lbs, and they couldn't wait to take me back home.

Our home at 62 Thornley Avenue was a two-bedroom council flat – what estate agents these days call an 'upper cottage flat' – in the west Glasgow suburb of Knightswood. My mother and father had moved there shortly after getting married in July 1939. For the next 55 years, until she moved into a nursing home for the last few months of her life, my mother never lived anywhere else. And as I never stopped visiting her there, and as it's where I spent the first 25 years of my own life, that house and Knightswood mattered to me a lot. It was my home, and I'm rather proud of the place.

Why? Because Knightswood, which was built in the 1920s, had been properly planned and thought-out, and the answers the planners had come up with chimed in with how people wanted to live their lives. They wanted shops, schools, libraries, churches and railway stations within easy walking distance, so even though they might be living at the edge of the city, it didn't feel like it. They wanted parks to play in, maybe even with a municipal golf course, pitch and putt greens and tennis courts attached, with the Campsie Fells on the horizon and the countryside just an easy walk or cycle-ride away. Most of all, when they moved out of the inner-city tenements to live there, they wanted their own patch of land too: a 10ft strip of garden in the front, with a waist-high hedge or curved iron railings to separate it from the pavement, and at the back a garden the size of a tennis court.

The estate on which the council built 6,174 houses was carved out of about four square miles of farmland and disused mining works just outside what was then the city's north-western boundary. All the flats had fitted bathrooms and decent-sized rooms – 'homes not hutches' in the words of John Wheatley, Labour's first Secretary of State for Health, whose 1924 Housing Act provided the financial guarantees councils needed to start building. But there was far more to the estate than that. It had eight churches, because this was still a rigorously Christian society. My parents were both devout members of the Church of Scotland and I grew up to share their faith. There were four shopping centres, each with enough for most families' daily needs, and six schools, both primary and secondary. At the end of our street there was even a library and a community centre.

Knightswood wasn't just the biggest housing estate Glasgow built between the wars, but it was arguably the best. On Saturday evenings, from 1939 to 1953, one of the most popular radio shows on the BBC's Scottish Home Service was a radio soap opera called *The McFlannels*. It was about a working-class Glasgow family who had originally lived in Partick tenements. When they moved to a four-room flat in Knightswood it was made quite clear that they had 'gone up in the world', although some of the characters complained that because it was so remote, commuting to work took too long.

Where we lived, though, that didn't seem so much of a problem. There was a good bus service, Scotstounhill railway station was only about a quarter of a mile away, and the nearest shipyard on Clyde was just about the same distance again. And when you reached the river, whether you looked left or right, for miles in either direction you'd see shipyards hard at work: great thickets of cranes at Barclay Curle, Charles Connell, Blythswood, Yarrow, Fairfield, and, a mile or so up the river, the famous John Brown yard at Clydebank, where they'd built the *Queen Mary* and where they would go on, after the war, to build her successors, the *Queen Elizabeth* and the *QE2*. In the early 1900s yards like these had produced a fifth of the world's ships. By the time of the Second World War, that proportion was falling back, but after the lean years of the Depression, the yards were busy again, and so were the other riverine businesses filleted between them: propeller and pump manufacturers, repair yards, engine works and dry docks. During the war, my father worked as an engineer in one of the Scotstoun shipyards. As this was a reserved occupation, he was exempt from conscription, though he also served in the Home Guard.

Sometimes, when I look back at my parents' photo albums from those days, it's hard to imagine that there ever was a war on. Certainly there are no signs of it in the pictures they took on holiday in Largs in June 1940. France might have fallen, and many people thought Britain might be next, but that wasn't going to stop Arthur and Grace Calman going on their first proper holiday after their honeymoon, walking down the promenade, watching films in the Viking Cinema, eating ice cream, and smiling for the camera. They were back in Largs again exactly a year later. The war was still going badly, but again there was no hint of that in the family photo album, just as there wasn't in the photographic record of their summer holiday in 1942, when we stayed in the Station House at Hopeman, on the Morayshire coast, after travelling to Inverness on the sleeper. By this time, I was six months old. My dad wrote a poem about me:

Six months ago on Christmas day
God filled our hearts with joy
He gave to us love's precious gift
A lovely baby boy
So Kenneth Charles we christened you
And will our vow fulfil
That with God's help your mum and dad
Will keep you from all ill

And yet the war was there, all the time, all around them. Even in those happy family snaps, it creeps in around the edges. Take my first appearance in the family album. It's 23 May 1942 and there I am, being proudly shown off to my adoring gran in our back garden. Again, at first glance, it seems as though it belongs in peacetime. But, look again at the garden and you can see that it has been given over to growing potatoes. By 1941, thanks to the Dig For Victory campaign, and the songs and recipe books of Captain Carrot and Potato Pete, Britain's food imports had halved to 14.65 million tonnes. Some 10,000 square miles of gardens and neglected spaces had been taken over by vegetable growers. At No. 62 Thornley Avenue, we were doing our bit too.

In some of the photographs, in the middle of the potatoes is the grim hump of an Anderson shelter. Again, there's nothing unusual about that. 2.1 million of these corrugated galvanised steel shelters were half-buried in Britain's gardens, with most resurrected in peacetime, as ours was, to serve as a garden shed where we also kept our bikes. But nine months before I was born, in the middle of the Clydebank Blitz the shelter had its use. I might even have been conceived in it!

On the night of 13 March 1941 the first of three waves of German bombers flew west over our house. They'd already done their aerial reconnaissance, and you can see the targets marked out on their large-scale (1cm:150m) briefing photographs. On them, Knightswood is unmarked, the neat geometry of its streets undisturbed by parked cars or indeed vehicles of any kind. The real targets were in Clydebank, just over a mile to the west. The giant Singer Sewing Machine works, then largely given over to munitions work (they made Sten guns), was the biggest one, but John Brown's shipyard wasn't far behind: this was, after all, where the British battle cruisers HMS *Hood* and HMS *Repulse* – both sunk, with appalling loss of life, later that year – had both been built. Beardmore's engineering works was badly hit, as were the Admiralty oil storage tanks at Kilpatrick, and a huge timber yard at Singer's was lost – the last two adding immeasurably to the fires that earlier incendiary bombs had started. Before the Clydebank Blitz there had been 12,000 houses in the town. Only seven were unscathed; 4,300 were destroyed or beyond repair. In the two-night bombing raids of 13 and 14 March 1941, 528 people died in the concentrated carnage of Clydebank, and a further 650 in Glasgow.[1]

It's odd, isn't it, the things you never ask your parents? While they were alive, I never remember asking either of them what it felt like as those German planes roared overhead under a full 'bomber's moon' and the Drumchapel ack-ack guns opened up – whether they were frightened and stayed in the Anderson shelter until the all-clear sirens sounded, or whether they couldn't stop themselves going outside to look at the flames devouring Clydebank. It wasn't as if they were far from the danger themselves. Some of the earliest bombs in the raid fell on Knightswood – on houses in Alderman Road, Baldric Road and Kestrel Road. But it was the eight foot-long cylindrical 1,000lb landmine that landed on Bankhead School that did the most damage. Witnesses reported hearing a 'flapping' sound, looking up and seeing it swing down by parachute, hitting the school roof, sliding down the slates and dropping down to the playground, where it exploded. The blast destroyed almost the whole of the west wing of Bankhead School, which at the time was being used as a first aid post, fire station and ARP (Air Raid Precaution) centre. Thirty-nine people were killed, including 21 auxiliary firefighters and two teenage messenger boys. The fire burnt until dusk the next evening. St David's, where we all went to church, was damaged in the raids too, but so slightly by comparison to the horrors at Bankhead School – which my brother Norman and I subsequently attended – that I can't remember anyone ever mentioning it.

People forget just how long the war overshadowed the peace that came in 1945. Norman was born that year, but even by the time he left Bankhead school in the mid-'50s, ten years after the end of the war and 15 years after the bombing, they still hadn't replaced the gym hall or the canteen. Rationing lasted almost as long: it only ended in 1954. Years later, when I was Chief Medical Officer for first Scotland and then England, I used to tell my political masters that if they really wanted a healthy population, they should bring it back. Britain's wartime diet may have been deeply unpopular, but the country has never had a healthier one.

That, then, is a snapshot of the place and the time I was born into. But before I got any further, I should introduce you to my parents and the rest of my family. I loved my Dad. I loved my Mum too, but she wasn't the one who played football with me in the back garden, put me on her shoulders to watch Rangers at Ibrox, taught me to play golf on Knightswood's municipal nine-hole course, or made wooden toys for me at Christmas. Dad was fun to be with, and he had a great sense of humour. He used to play a game called Mr Bumble, where he dressed up and sang, 'My name is Bobbie Bumble, he doesn't mind a tumble, but up he jumps, and rubs his bumps and doesn't even grumble' and fell on the floor. It always made me laugh anyway. After the war, when work started to dry up in the shipyards, he got a job as a mechanic at MacKinnon's, a local textile manufacturer. I always looked forward to seeing him. To this day, I can remember listening out for him as he walked home along the street, whistling the first few bars of the *Woody Woodpecker* theme tune.

He was the youngest of eight children (and two who didn't survive childhood) and as all of them had children of their own, I had plenty of Calman cousins. The one I never knew was Charles, who was killed by the Japanese on the day I was born. He was the son of my uncle Alex, who had moved out to Hong Kong, where he managed a shipyard. I never knew my paternal grandfather either, but he was the one who brought the family from Dundee, where they lived at Lochee, to Glasgow early in the previous century. The word Calman is Gaelic and means a dove or pigeon, and the family, and the name, have an interesting history.[2] They lived in Partick, a district in Glasgow near the Clyde. My father attended Hamilton Crescent School, which he left when he was 14 to work in the shipyards. I have a Certificate of Merit for him from his final year, where his subjects included Laws of Health, Civics and the Empire.

My mother's family were also very close to me. She had been born Grace Douglas Don and her sister Cathy lived close by in Knightswood with her family and my Gran Daisy. Her brother and his family lived for a long time in the South Ayrshire village of Dailly, near Girvan. At one time he had a chip shop in which I occasionally helped out: not bad training for a future Chief Medical Officer! My father's brother, Charles, and his family also lived in Ayrshire: he was a Hoover salesman with great patter and his key phrase when going anywhere was 'The sky's the limit!' His daughter Doreen had a special dance which she demonstrated at weddings to the tune of 'Salome' with great effect.

Mum was devoted to my father. She wasn't as much of an extrovert as him, and if you didn't know her you might even mark her down as being quite shy, but they seemed to complement each other. She had been secretary to Sir Hugh (later Lord) Fraser and was an excellent typist and typed my PhD thesis. Her mother lived in Knightswood along with her sister, my auntie Cathy, so there was plenty of family support on hand to help in bringing up me and my brother Norman. Beyond the family, there was the church and the Women's Guild, and, after the war, the community centre at the end of our street, where she won prizes for her baking, sewing, and special tablet – a wonderful fudge. She loved the cinema too, and would regularly head off with my father to catch the latest shows at the Ascot, the Rosevale and the Vogue. My bedroom was just across the hall from the sitting room, and I can still remember crawling there like Wee Willie Winkie, unable to sleep and wanting a story, as my babysitters Moira and Norma sat on the sofa in front of a coal fire banked with dross, ready to last through till morning.

I've always been a hoarder, so I've held onto quite a number of things from my childhood that I hardly remember or don't remember at all. My mother's baby book, for example, informs me that I first slept through the night aged ten months, and that I started walking about the same time. By 18 months, I could say 'Please, mummy', 'Thanks' and (very polite) 'Pardon me'. On Monday 10 February 1947, I first went to school, and apparently liked it. My dad made me a wooden rocking chair, in which I was photographed when I was one. I've still got it, and my children and grandchildren have sat in it, just like I still have the three cut-down hickory golf clubs he used to teach me on the nine-hole Knightswood municipal course (threepence for children on Tuesday and Thursday afternoons). I still remember the sign on the clubhouse, 'Each player must have at least 3 clubs, one of which must be a putter'. When I was eight, and we were on a family holiday in St Andrews, the two of us played all three major courses, including the Old Course, which probably isn't possible to do now. I've also still got my father's helmet and booklet from his Home Guard days, bits of blackout material, the airplane hangar he made me for Christmas in the war when toys were luxuries beyond compare. I can tell you that when I saw the Scottish Cup Final on 20

May 1944, I sat in Section K, Row L, on the East Stand, though I can't tell you anything else about the game. And the first time I saw Rangers play a foreign side was on 25 November the following year, when they played Moscow Dynamos – who caused controversy by taking to the field with 12 players. It was a Wednesday afternoon kick-off, but still a stonking 10 shillings a ticket.

Without anything I've hoarded to prompt my memory, however, I can still remember the big freeze in 1947, when the snows were so deep that the Great Western Road – the A82, the main road to Loch Lomond – was closed, and we could sledge down a hill and all the way across it. And I can remember Hogmanay in the days when the Clyde was rammed with ships, and the sound of their horns at midnight welcomed in the New Year. In 1948, I remember the huge family reunion we had in Troon, when uncle Alex and his wife Laura finally came back to Scotland from the Far East. He had been captured after the fall of Hong Kong in which his son had been killed, and spent the rest of the war in appalling conditions in Japanese prisoner of war camps. By the time peace came, he was completely emaciated, and had no idea what had happened to his wife: mercifully, she had somehow managed to escape to Australia, where they finally met up again.

Significant or trivial, but all mixed together – that's how memories flood back when I reflect on my childhood. Firing up the memory neurons in my brain, a whole variety of unrelated scenes and facts from childhood leap across my synapses. My mother tying my laces and asking me to run down and see what food was in the shops ('There's mince in the butcher's' I would announce to the whole street on those comparatively rare days when there was). Long games of marbles that we'd play on roads empty of all traffic apart from the occasional horse-drawn coal cart. Listening to *Children's Hour* on the radio. Cycling for a picnic in the Bluebell Woods of (then undeveloped) Drumchapel. Playing interminable games of football where we used the 'pig-bins' (where food waste was kept to be fed to pigs: another hangover from wartime rationing) as goal-posts. Long after I ever needed to know it, I can recite my Co-op number – 251214 – or the best-ever Rangers line-up (Brown, Young, Shaw, McColl, Woodburn, Cox, Waddell, Gillick, Thornton, Finlay and Duncanson). Shards of my childhood are buried in memories like that, or in the print of the football programmes I used to collect, or in the pages of the ten volumes of Arthur Mee's *Children's Encyclopedia*, which I was given for my seventh birthday.

But there's one memory from my childhood that overshadows all others. On 25 June 1951, Norman was looking out of the window hoping to see Dad coming whistling up the street when he saw a policeman opening our gate. Seconds later there was a knock on our main door, at the side of the house. Mum went down and he told her that she'd better get round to the Western Infirmary, because my dad had just been taken there. She ordered Norman and me to go out and play and went off to find Mr Kirkland, one of only two people in our street who had a car, to ask if he'd take her to the hospital.

We were playing football in the next street a couple of hours or so later when one of the neighbours came to find us and told us that we were wanted back home. He didn't say why, but I knew there was something wrong as soon as I turned the corner. There were three cars, all parked outside our house. Norman, being only six, didn't realise that spelt trouble. The two of us went up the stairs and into the lounge. It was packed out with relatives: Mum's sister, Auntie Cathy and her mum, our Gran, had walked over from Upper Knightswood. On my father's side, Auntie Dove and Uncle Tec had driven over from Newlands, Auntie Jean and Uncle Jimmy had come from Baillieston and Aunt Ellen and Uncle Willie from Rutherglen. They all looked up at us with pity in their eyes. I forget who it was who told us that my father had just died of a heart attack.

Dad had been to see the doctor that morning about something quite trivial – a painful toe that was probably gout. Yet as he was being examined, he had symptoms of a heart attack. The GP told him he should go straight to hospital. He took a bus to Western Infirmary, where he collapsed and died at the porter's gate. He was just 41.

* * *

For most of my life since that day, I've wondered what it would take to make a heavy smoker like my father stop. When I was Chief Medical Officer, working out an answer to that question, that would apply to everyone, was a key part of my job. How do you stop someone smoking? Is spelling out the risks enough or will smokers just ignore the mountainous accretion of evidence that it's bad for them? At what point do you give up on efforts to try to persuade them – or should you? What, in short, works? And would it have worked for Dad? That's one of the biggest 'what if' questions in my life – and if anything, it has grown even bigger in my mind as I have grown older. As the years have gone by, I actually miss my father more and more. I think of the joy my wife Ann and I have found watching our grandchildren Grace and Brodie grow up. I know he would have felt that same delight in our own children – Andrew, Lynn and Susan.

My father had died only a year after the first definitive evidence of the link between smoking and lung cancer emerged.[3] Smoking was not only socially acceptable, but, hard as it is to understand now, the first government information campaigns actually encouraged it. In 1917, the Pipes and Tobacco League sent tobacco to soldiers and sailors on the frontline, arguing that it was good for their health as well as for morale. Six million men who served in the First World War were introduced to smoking when they joined up, and free tobacco only encouraged their addiction. Such attitudes carried on into the Second World War public health education too: a wartime 'Blood donors wanted' poster featured an injured soldier being tended by his comrades while contentedly drawing on a cigarette. The 1947 Budget even went so far as issuing pensioners with tobacco vouchers to offset tax increases.[4]

Back then, of course, I knew nothing about any of this, or that this was one of the main directions my life would take. I was just a nine-year-old boy shattered by grief. I now have close on 70 years of hindsight, and I occasionally think of how easy it would be for that nine-year-old boy's world to collapse. But it didn't. We were surrounded, I can now see, by love. It was there in my primary school teachers (Miss Bissell and Miss McKellar), despite having classes of 50-plus to contend with, taking the time to encourage me. I knew they cared. When school ended on my first day back, one of them came to me, bent down and did up the buttons of my coat. She'd never done that before – no teacher had – but as she did, I saw tears welling in her eyes.

And it wasn't just her. In searching through my archives, I came across a small autograph book. The biggest cluster of contributions to it from friends and relatives came in July and August 1951 and include signatures they knew would mean a lot to me, like those from Rangers and Queen's Park football players. It's as if my family, friends and neighbours were trying to take my mind off my father's death and giving me other things to think about. We had always been a close family, and my father's death didn't change that: his family always remained close and supportive, just as my mother's did.

Then there was the community centre, less than 100 yards away at the end of our street. After it opened in 1950, it was where about 20 or 30 of us would go in the years before we had a television of our own, to sit in front of the 12-inch screen and watch programmes like *What's My Line?*. Communal television-watching was then fairly commonplace, as it was only after the Queen's coronation that we, along with millions of other families, got a set of our own. We watched the coronation on the tiny set hired for the day and placed in the church hall at St David's. We had packed sandwiches and taken them to church, where the minister had led a special coronation service before we went into the church hall to watch events at Westminster Abbey. In my surprisingly neat 11-year-old's copperplate, I wrote up what happened next:

We saw our beautiful Queen Elizabeth crowned. As well as seeing the television, we got sweets, balloons, lemonade and tea. At night, we went round the parks watching the fireworks and seeing bonfires. At last we had to go home, but what a lovely day it had been.

Generally, though, it was at the community centre that most of our social life took place. They held Scottish country dancing classes there, and there was a room in which Miss John's Orchestra rehearsed (with me on drums: my favourite was *The Radetzsky March* by Johann Strauss). There was a library there too, and both my mother and I used it a lot: her to borrow romantic novels, me to work my way through books like Enid Blyton's *Famous Five* series or Angus MacVicar's *The Lost Planet*. Before the war, there had been plans to build a swimming pool there too, but the council had run out of money and the site was fenced off. This – along with the fact that it was a shortcut between our house and Bankhead primary school half a mile away and that we could easily climb over the fence – meant that the long-abandoned building site became our unofficial adventure playground.

My father's death meant that looking after the garden now became my responsibility, and as I grew older and stronger I used to help out with neighbour's gardens too, which provided me with a bit of pocket money. While I was at school I used to help my uncle, who made and repaired watches and clocks, for a couple of afternoons each week. Usually, this involved taking repaired watches to the shops, or doing odd jobs. Sometimes, however, I cleaned the clocks and began the process of rebuilding and resetting them. It was fascinating, and to this day my brother Norman keeps the small business going. For me, however, the key thing was my interest in time; how important it was and how it should not be wasted – something I still feel strongly. It also underlies my interest in sundials, which continues to this day. I had plenty of hobbies – making balsa wood model aeroplanes, stamp collecting, and photography among them – but my real priorities were elsewhere: church and the Boys' Brigade, music and study.

It is hard to underestimate how important Christianity has been to me, not only now, but in my teenage years too. Even when my father was alive I'd attended Sunday school, and later joined the Scripture Union, went to their camps, and won a Young Worshippers' League prize for attending a Sunday service every week for five years. St David's was close to our home and its Christmas Eve midnight service still lingers in my memory – and not just because my birthday started when it ended. At midnight, as we sang 'Still the Night', the lights were dimmed and left only the cross lit up with a star on a dark blue velvet curtain background.

The church always had a series of powerful ministers, and the one I remember most was the Reverend Eric Alexander, who was at St David's for four years before going on to be minister at St George's Tron church in the centre of the city. I saw him as a role model, and even briefly contemplated being a minister. In April 1955, I had, after all, seen the most impressive evangelist in the world. The first night Billy Graham preached at the Kelvin Hall, on 21 March 1955, 16,000 people turned up. 'But when I gave the Invitation at the end of the sermon,' Graham said afterwards, 'not a soul moved. I bowed my head in prayer, and moments later, when I looked up, people were streaming down the aisles, some with tears in their eyes.'[5] It's hard these days to convey the effect Billy Graham had on Scotland that year. Even the statistics, though verifiable, seem completely implausible now: audiences of 2,647,365 people in the entire All Scotland Crusade, church attendances in Glasgow 50 per cent higher at the end of the decade than before he arrived, 100,000 people at his farewell rally at Hampden (and, in those more ordered and respectful days, not a single one of them on the pitch), a worldwide audience of 30 million for his Good Friday rally at Kelvin Hall. But those figures don't even begin to explain what it felt like to watch, as I did, Billy Graham's rally at Kelvin Hall. This was, remember, the biggest exhibition hall in Europe, and it was packed. Packed with people who hung on the preacher's every word, whose lives were changed by his message. I was already sure of my Christian faith, but that Kelvin Hall rally had a profound effect on me all the same.

All through my teenage years, the Boys' Brigade was a hugely important part of my life. 'The best way to enjoy yourself in the Life Boys,' the membership card of its junior branch advised, 'is to put your heart into everything.' I did too, moving up into the Boys' Brigade proper and then ascending the ranks until I was 18, when I was a staff sergeant. (Years later that ascent continued, as I became first President of the Glasgow Battalion and then UK President of the Brigade in 2007. Little did I know that my future wife, Ann, was also heavily involved in the organisation.)

The Boys' Brigade's Glasgow credentials are impeccable (it was founded there in 1883 by Sir William Smith), but for me it had many other attractions. Its Friday meetings were where my folk singing began and my limited acting talents found their first stage. Working towards the various badges – woodwork, birdwatching and so on – they taught me practical skills I might not have acquired anywhere else. For my first aid, I learned to master the basic skills of bandaging and resuscitation, and although I never thought so at the time, in hindsight that might have been the first glimmer of an interest in a career in medicine.

But of course, I didn't think like that. The 14-year-old corporal in his Boys' Brigade pillbox cap, assiduously learning about marching and playing the drums in its pipe band (for which Norman played the bagpipes) didn't have a clue what career he wanted to pursue. I followed the old Life Boy mantra and put my heart into everything they taught me, and ended up as the troop's best-drilled recruit and winner of the trophy for 'best all-round boy'. I mightn't have known what I wanted to do with my life at that stage, but the Boys' Brigade gave me a sense of purpose. Its motto of 'Sure and steadfast' could just as easily have been mine too: I shared its Christian values and aims ('the advancement of Christ's kingdom among Boys and the promotion of habits of obedience, reverence, discipline self-respect and all that tends towards a true Christian manliness') and looked forward to the Bible study sessions that were every bit as important a part of our Sundays as were the parades. These were, as Billy Graham's crusade made clear, different days: stronger in Christian faith than our own. Where St David's had six Boys' Brigades squads in my time, there now isn't even one.

During the week, I wore another uniform: the navy blazer of Allan Glen's. This was a remarkable school, founded in the middle of the 19th century by a successful Glasgow businessman who left an endowment 'to give a good practical education and preparation for trades or businesses, to between forty to fifty boys, the sons of tradesmen or persons in the industrial classes of society'. It did a lot more than that. Over the years, it established a reputation as being Scotland's best school for teaching science, and the roll call of its eminent former pupils would prove the point. One of the most famous was the architect Charles Rennie Macintosh, and when I first started thinking seriously about my career, I thought that I might try to follow in his footsteps.

At Allan Glen's I developed a great interest in science and technology, as might be expected. But the arts were also important to me, especially music, and I sang in the school choir. Through one of my longstanding friends, Andrew Dobson, I was introduced to classical music and bought my first records, *Finlandia* by Sibelius and Beethoven's Violin Concerto. Andrew and I keep in touch and he still sends me terrible jokes. Painting was also important at school, as was pottery, woodwork and metalwork. I loved making things. This was also when I wrote, in neat italic handwriting, and then bound my first book, 'The History of Flight'. I still have it at home.

Although I had won a bursary to Allan Glen's, money was still tight – in fact, there wasn't any coming into the house apart from a small widow's pension. So my mother began to take in boarders, two at a time, who were training to be physical education teachers at the nearby Jordanhill College. She replaced her double bed with two singles and the two students took over that bedroom. Norman and I shared the other one. Mum slept on a pull-down bed in the lounge. When I look back and think of what she did for us all, as a single mother bringing up two young boys, I am overcome with gratitude.

The only problem was that our two-bedroom flat was completely full. There wasn't anywhere for me to do my homework. After making us all a meal, in the evening mum would put her feet up in front of the television. The students would either work in their own room or join her in the lounge. Either way, there wasn't anywhere else I could get out my books and study. But I wasn't going to be put off easily. To the right at the top of our stairs, between the bedroom and the lounge, there was a small cupboard space. Technically, it was a walk-in cupboard, because it had a door and you could walk in, although it was only four-foot deep and little more than the width of the door. There was a waist-high shelf at which I could sit and, using it as a desk, spread out my books while everyone's coats and jackets hung on hooks behind me. There was just one drawback; the walk-in cupboard didn't have an electric light, so I used candles placed in a tin box. And that is where it all began, my learning and writing, both of which have brought me great happiness.

I have kept all my school exercise books, along with timetables, reading lists and even exam papers for my 1959 Scottish Higher Leaving Certificate (I'd find them impossible to do now). And as I take them out of their box, glance at the school's coat of arms (two compasses above a set square) on the cover, I find it easy to imagine the years dissolving and being back at 62 Thornley Avenue, my younger self beginning to learn the basics of chemistry, calculus, trigonometry or dynamics in the soft, flickering candlelight.[6]

Allan Glen's widened my horizons in other ways too – sometimes painfully. Rugby was the sport of choice at school, and my height (or lack of it: 5ft 3¾ins is the tallest I've been) meant that I was a natural pick as a hooker. In those days, the rules for scrums were different, and hookers were allowed to swing forward and into the opposition pack to retrieve the ball. I was reasonably good at this, though I did have some accidents, and my nose was broken twice. While I was struggling with my rugby, my cousin Jimmy Docherty (JT Docherty) was being picked to play for Scotland. In 1955, in his second match, he scored a drop-goal in the 14-8 victory over Wales at Murrayfield.[7] His father, another Jimmy, who married my father's sister, had the distinction of playing football for both Rangers and Celtic. Like my own father, my cousin died much too young.

Even before I went to Allan Glen's, at weddings and other family gatherings, I'd often be dragged out to sing songs such as 'Over the Sea to Skye' or 'If I Can Help Somebody'. I also became interested in folk music, both Scottish and American, and decided to learn the guitar. I couldn't afford to buy one, so I made one from a kit. I played skiffle music with a group at the Boys' Brigade and expanded my folk repertoire by cutting out and learning the learning the songs published each week in the *Glasgow Bulletin* newspaper. My hero was Lonnie Donegan.

What with music, sport, the Boys' Brigade and homework, my teenage years at school were satisfyingly busy. But as I moved into my last year, I still hadn't got a clear idea of what career path I should be aiming at. And here my memory, normally so clear, lets me down. All I remember is that the Calman cousins were having one of our regular get-togethers when the subject came up. I can't remember who was there, or whose house we were in, only that I told them I was thinking about studying engineering.

'Really?' said one of my older cousins. 'What about medicine? Have you ever thought of that?'

Everyone else in the room seemed to think it was a good idea. Why, I don't know. It wasn't as though there were any doctors in our family and I didn't even know anyone who was one. Against that, at Allan Glen's I'd had as good a secondary education as any working-class Scot could hope for. I'd worked hard and conscientiously. So why not?

CHAPTER 2

The Tram from St George's Cross

I SOMETIMES TELL people that I got my wife off the back of a lorry, and it's not a word of a lie. Towards the end of January 1960, Glasgow students were planning their annual Charities Day Parade. Although the tradition has died out now, back then it was a huge carnival – an 'invasion' of the city centre in which lorries were turned into carnival floats and packed with students in fancy dress shaking collecting cans in shoppers' faces. As well as the lorries, there would be a surreal march-past of pipe bands, followed by students dressed in homemade costumes as knights, ghosts, animals and clowns. The parade would wend its way through the city centre towards a viewing platform where it was inspected by the university's Charities Queen, sometimes with the Lord Provost in attendance. As it passed, onlookers would lob pennies at the passing floats or put coins in the students' collecting tins.

Back then, I was playing banjo in an eight-piece jazz band, having moved on from the guitar. This made sense: musically, because these were the days of Louis Armstrong, Sidney Bechet, and the Clyde Valley Stompers; financially, because we were paid the heady sum of ten shillings a night. One of the boys in the band was going out with a girl who was a trainee teacher at Jordanhill College. For Charities Day on 30 January, she and her friends decided that they wanted to dress up as flappers and dance the Charleston on the back of a lorry that would join the big parade to George Square before peeling off to collect money in the suburbs. They needed us to provide the music as they danced round the city. First, though, the lorry had to be decorated with streams of coloured paper, they had to meet us, and we had to rehearse.

So that's why, in a lorry depot at the bottom of University Avenue on 29 January 1960, I met the woman who would become my wife.

'Are you one of the dancers?' I asked hopefully.

'Yes. Who are you?'

'I'm in the band.'

We introduced ourselves. She was called Ann. I don't know what she made of me, but at least, in my university blazer and scarf, I was looking smart.

The next morning we all got on the back of the lorry and waited for the parade to start. To be honest, I've seen better floats, but none of the girls had that much money so the lorry wasn't going to turn into, for example, a papier-mâché battleship. The theme they'd decided on was 'Stairway to Heaven', but the only stairs were a couple of step-ladders, and the only heaven was – well, I guess it was meant to be the eight Jordanhill girls shimmying on the back of a flatbed lorry in their beaded pink 'flapper' dresses.

The parade set off from Kelvin Way, and Ann and the seven other Jordanhill girls started dancing – to keep themselves warm as much as anything. We turned left into Argyll Street, where the crowds grew bigger the nearer we got to the city centre. As we trundled along, we worked through our repertoire: 'When the Saints Go Marching In', 'Tiger Rag', 'Just A Little While to Stay Here', 'Muskrat Ramble', 'The Charleston' and 'Marching Through Georgia'. The Jordanhill girls danced, the collectors shouted 'Phil McCann!' and rattled their collecting tins under people's noses, and the lorry moved ever nearer George Square. In one respect, it was a good day for a parade: neither Celtic nor Rangers were playing at home, so there'd be more men around to put money in the collecting tins. On the other hand, it was even colder than you'd expect from a January morning in Glasgow. I was wearing a coat and hat and was still trying not to shiver: for the girls in their short, thin dresses, it must have been even worse. It was so cold that I couldn't feel my hands, and it was a while before I noticed that I'd been pressing down so hard on the strings with my fingers that there was blood on the banjo.

That night, though, we all went dancing at the students' union. By the end of the night, Ann and I had paired off, and I had forgotten about the cold altogether. For a few years after this I continued to play in the band, at the interval at the University Union on Saturday nights, and at various local venues, and on at least one occasion I played my banjo with the visiting band, The Clyde Valley Stompers – the pinnacle of my musical career!

* * *

I loved Ann, but I loved learning too. Almost everything about medicine was new to me, but that was a challenge, not a curse. If our family wasn't the kind that routinely produced doctors, didn't that make becoming one that little bit more special? If I knew next to nothing about how hospitals worked, wasn't it going to be just that little bit more interesting to find out? If I had never studied biology at school, how was that going to hold me back when I already had so many other new subjects to cram into my brain? There is a word for people like me who have a passion for acquiring new knowledge. We are *philomaths*. And when you are a medical student, it doesn't half help if you are one. There are, you soon discover, quite a few subjects to master: anatomy, physiology, pharmacology, pathology, bacteriology, medicine, surgery, dermatology, obstetrics and gynaecology, forensic medicine, venereal diseases, paediatrics, psychiatry, general practice, ENT (ear, nose and throat) ophthalmology, public health and lots more, each one with class exams and certificates.

Even that, though, wasn't enough for me. During my third year as a medical student I was invited, along with a few others, to spend what would have been my fourth and fifth years studying for an extra science degree. Universities call this an 'intercalated' degree, which basically means a second degree sandwiched between the first one, which you then go back and finish. On the plus side, because I was already studying medicine, the science degree would take two years rather than four. On the minus side, a medicine degree at the time took a full six years, so adding on another two was a substantial commitment. My mother, for one, couldn't understand why I would want to do it. And then there was Ann. We knew we were serious about each other early on. If I did do another degree, it would be another two years before we could get married. How was that fair on her?

Actually, when I asked what she thought, she couldn't have been more supportive. It was at that moment, she says, that she realised two things about me. She had always thought I'd got a good sense of humour, but this was when she understood that I was serious about wanting to do as much as I could with my life, and how this meant learning as much as I could too. Without Ann, I couldn't have done half the things I have done in my life. She has been the best partner imaginable. I'd no idea that the girl dancing the Charleston in front of me on the back of a lorry would ever mean so much to me. That's something else I have learnt too.

Memories of my life as a medical student are inseparable from memories of Ann. As I got to know her, I came to know and enjoy the company of her family too. Her parents lived in St George's Cross, near the centre of town. Her father was a talented silversmith who worked as an engineer in Barr & Stroud's during the war making periscopes and navigational instruments. He was a well-known long-distance runner with the Maryhill Harriers but, like my own father, died far too young, in 1963. When Ann and I got engaged on Christmas Eve the following year, it was a source of regret that neither of our fathers were there to be part of the celebrations.

By then, though, we had amassed many happier memories together. For me, those included watching Ann as Puck in her college's production of *A Midsummer Night's Dream*, and the Daft Friday Ball held at the end of each first term (for which she made her own ballgowns – yet another of her many talents). We spent holidays in Montrose, where she had relatives, and in 1964 made the first of what has turned out to be many visits to Arran, with Ann riding pillion on my Tiger Cub motorbike.

I often think back to my courting days, and when I do I have a memory which is almost like a recurring dream. In it, I am coming back on the last tram from St George's Cross to Knightswood. The trams are long gone now – 4 September, 1962 was their last day – but they carry on rattling up the Great Western Road in my imagination. I'm on board, sitting at the front, and behind me I can hear friendly late-night Glaswegian banter. It matches my own good mood. Sometimes my imagination adds a thick, swirling fog outside the window – and that's something else that, thanks to the 1956 Clean Air Act, doesn't happen now, or hardly ever. In the early '60s, though, those kinds of fogs were a regular enough occurrence in Glasgow. On the

No 10 bus home from university it wasn't unusual for a passenger to get out and walk in front of the bus because the driver couldn't see a thing. I've done it myself on more than one occasion. Ann remembers fogs so thick that the buses stopped running altogether. Coming home from school she had to feel her way along Kelvinbridge (the cast iron bridge over the River Kelvin on the Great Western Road) because she couldn't see more than a couple of feet in front of her.

Back to the intercalated degree. When, with Ann's backing, I decided that I would like to do one, I opted to study biochemistry. The discovery of the structure of DNA less than a decade earlier had made this a 'hot' subject, but to master it I had also to do extra chemistry, learn about statistics and do courses in French and German, the two languages of science.[1] Plenty, in other words, to keep my inner philomath happy. Without a state grant, of course, all of this would have been impossible. My research interests were supervised by Dr Hamish Keir, another mentor, who subsequently became a professor at Aberdeen University. One of the features of the university at this time was that every medical student had a tutor who mentored a small group. I was fortunate in having Mr Willie Mack, a urologist, as mine. For someone like myself, with no medical background, it was invaluable to have someone to talk to and guide me. He and Mrs Mack were delightful hosts and I have much to thank them for.

Looking back, I suppose this was one of my first steps away from a more-travelled academic path. There's a hint of why I took it in one of my favourite quotes. In his 1859 book *The Professor at the Breakfast Table*, Oliver Wendell Holmes writes the following:

> The longer I live, the more I am satisfied of two things: first, that the truest lives are those that are cut rose-diamond fashion, with many facets, answering to the many planed surfaces of the world about them: secondly, that society is always trying in some way or another to grind us down to a single flat surface.

I have always thought this a particularly apposite quote in relation to the doctor-patient encounter and how the patient should never be seen as merely as a collection of symptoms in need of a solution. Indeed, as we shall soon see, my own medical education was lit up by people who always emphasised the importance of treating patients as more than a collection of bones, muscles and cells but as a whole person, with feelings and anxieties waiting to be listened to and understood. But Holmes's message can, I think, also apply to medics' minds too: and in studying biochemistry, I was just trying to make my own mind a bit more multifaceted, not least in relation to cutting-edge science.

The purpose of medical education, in one sense, is obvious – to prepare a person with the skills, knowledge and values to practice as a doctor. However, there is a deeper purpose, preparing a person for a life devoted to caring for others. During the time in medical school there is an opportunity to consider this purpose and, if necessary, decide not to pursue a career in medicine. After I had been accepted to study medicine at Glasgow University, I looked around for books to read, and found some in a now defunct bookshop in central Glasgow. On my way home, I walked up the High Street to the Cathedral, where the university began in 1451 in St Mungo's Crypt. The university was established on the model of the University of Bologna, and the Papal Bull which established it had the following wonderful phrase:

> That there may be an overflowing fountain of the sciences out of whose fullness all that desire to be imbued with the lessons of knowledge may drink.

As part of my degree I had to complete a short research-based thesis. Both doing that and working on a Carnegie research scholarship in the two summer holidays, I came to realise the attractions of research science. The work I did as a demonstrator in the medical student laboratory classes also further encouraged my interest in teaching. Of those two interests, it was research that at first seemed to be getting the upper hand.

During the biochemistry course, I had met Dr John Milne, one of Scotland's leading dermatologists and soon to be appointed to the university's first chair in the subject. I had been working on a project about the sebaceous gland – essentially to see whether it could be persuaded to stop producing acne – and we had spent a summer in Finland researching skin histochemistry on a Wellcome scholarship. When I went back to being a medical student in 1965, he suggested that I should turn the project into a PhD. It took me five years, part of which was as a medical student. The other research interest I had was with Mr John Hamilton, a consultant orthopaedic surgeon who was experimenting with new hip prostheses. Gordon Waddell, another student in my year, was also part of the project and he went on to become an outstanding orthopaedic consultant.

Perhaps, I might now concede, all of this was carrying philomathy a bit too far. For one thing, in the two years in which I had been studying biochemistry, the medicine degree had been shortened from six years to five. This was good news – one year less before Ann and I could get married – but it meant that I had more to catch up on, not least a whole lecture course I had missed on medicine and surgery. As well as reading up on that, I was doing the normal year four and year five work for my medicine degree. Those years, and the years spent training to be a surgeon, are generally – rightly – held to be particularly demanding. Yet on top of all that work, and starting my married life with Ann (we were married on 8 July, 1967) I had also to finish my PhD. No wonder I never seemed to have any spare time.

But I am getting ahead of myself. Let me move back from the work-filled weekends and stresses of being a trainee surgeon in the late-1960s and take you back to the start of the decade and my very first weeks as a medical student. Because it was then that I learnt one of the most important lessons of my life in medicine. And it is a lesson I can sum up in just one word. For that word, though, we have to go a lot further back – all the way to 7 March 161AD, and join the Emperor Antoninus Pius at his palace in Lorium, 12 miles west of Rome, on the last day of his life. He was 75, and his 23-year reign as emperor was one of the most beneficent in Roman history, a time of peace (apart from a small war against the rebellious Scots) and prosperity. Realising that he was dying, he summoned his imperial council and made all of the arrangements necessary for a smooth transfer of power. When the captain of the guard came to ask what the password for the night should be, he gave a one-word answer that not only summed up his philosophy of life but was also the last thing he said. '*Aequanimitas*,' he said. Equanimity.

I first came across that story in a book I'd bought in my first year studying medicine. *Aequanimitas* is the title of a 1904 book of essays and speeches by Sir William Osler that is widely regarded as a classic of medical literature. In it Osler (1849–1919), a Canadian who went on to become the first Professor of the renowned Johns Hopkins Medical School in Baltimore and Regius Professor of Medicine at Oxford, argues that the key quality to which any clinician should aspire is imperturbability – the ability to maintain one's equilibrium while dealing with the devastation of disease on others and also with one's own personal problems. Such composure, he argues, is essential, especially when treating impressionable or frightened patients. This, he said, was 'a bodily virtue': some people have it, others don't. But its mental equivalent, he added, citing the story of Antoninus Pius's last word, was *aequanimitas*. Equanimity was something all doctors should try to cultivate and the best ones would succeed. Osler wrote his essay in 1889, six years before Kipling opened his poem 'If' with a textbook definition of equanimity ('If you can keep your head when all about you/Are losing theirs'), but its message in a medical context was clear: no matter what the situation, how bad the emergency, doctors should remain calm, attentive, sympathetic and in control of the situation. One of Osler's fellow-doctors at Johns Hopkins, noted that he practised what he preached. 'Many who came in contact with him,' he wrote, 'never realised how much anxiety he often felt but rarely displayed over patients.'[2] Osler, who is sometimes called 'the father of modern medicine', is one of my great heroes. At Johns Hopkins, he was one of the first to insist that medical students accompany him on his hospital rounds. He emphasised the importance of them learning to take down detailed patient histories ('Listen to your patient, he is telling you the diagnosis') and pioneered the practice of bedside teaching.

The other set of books that I discovered at the time were three volumes of *Horae Subsecivae* by Dr John Brown, an Edinburgh doctor. It is a series of short stories and my favourite is 'Rab and his Friends'. This is the story, first published in 1859, of a woman called Ailie who develops a lump in her breast, has seen the surgeon and agrees to undergo a mastectomy. It is narrated by a medical student who escorts the patient into theatre where she is also accompanied by her husband and Rab the dog. The operating theatre is full of medical students watching the operation. The key to the story is that the operation is performed before the introduction of anaesthesia by James Young Simpson in Edinburgh. Ailie bows to the students, lies down, and the operation is performed. At the end she comes down from the table, curtsies to the students and begs their pardon. They are all in tears. She leaves the theatre with Rab and her husband. The effect of this story on me was significant and began my interest in the link between literature and medicine and the lessons we can learn.

Glasgow has its own pantheon of medical greats, and they have left their mark all over the city. If, for example, I was going to my first-term anatomy class, I would catch the train in from home to Charing Cross and walk past Woodside Place, where Joseph Lister, the pioneer of antiseptic surgery, once lived. (He performed the first operation using antisepsis in the city's Royal Infirmary, which also, thanks to the work of John Macintyre, had the world's first radiology unit.) Then I'd walk through Kelvingrove Park past the memorial fountain to Robert Stewart (admittedly not a medic, but his work in providing the city with water from Loch Katrine was also a life-saver) to the university, where the library was just below the Hunterian Museum (founded by the eminent Glasgow-trained 18th-century anatomist and obstetrician William Hunter). The medical school had already produced so many innovative clinicians, from George Beatson's pioneering work on breast cancer to Ian Donald's breakthrough in ultrasound.

With his groundbreaking work on duodenal ulcers, Sir Andrew Kay, the Regius Professor of Surgery who taught me in my fourth and fifth years, was firmly in that league. Many people have an image of surgeons as loud, arrogant males (in those days, they mainly *were* males) who disregard their staff and all but ignore their patients. Some are indeed like that, but that wasn't the kind of surgeon I ever wanted to be. Sir Andrew Kay was a much better role model: a surgeon who never forgot that the patient is a real person with feelings and concerns, not just a collection of symptoms to be analysed. I wish you could have seen him, as I have, examining the abdomen of a young boy in acute pain. It was the perfect embodiment of what Osler means by *aequanimitas*. Kay was consistently gentle, always watching the patient respond, always explaining what he was doing and why, even when he pressed firmer, constantly gauging the patient's reaction until he found the diagnosis. To see this was not to forget it.

Here, at the patient's bedside, was a practical demonstration of the 'clinical method' – the process by which, in a systematic way, the story is listened to, further questions pursued, clinical examination carried out, investigations undertaken and a provisional diagnosis made. This is always done with full cooperation with the patient and consideration is then given to possible treatment. I have used this method in other spheres of life to understand a problem, undertake specialist reviews and investigations, and come up with a possible solution. But what Sir Andrew was demonstrating wasn't just technique, it was the knowledge and expertise he had gathered in all his years as a gastroenterologist that allowed him to make the diagnosis in the first place.

We only had the privilege of watching Sir Andrew at work by the time we were in our fourth year. A medical degree is a staged accumulation of knowledge, and without already possessing a detailed knowledge of anatomy, and other subjects, we wouldn't have been able to profitably learn from his example. But for more than two years most of our days had started off with anatomy classes, in which we gathered, six to a table, to learn the intricacies of the human body by dissecting one. As groups were arranged alphabetically, I got to know my fellow-students whose names begin with the letter 'C' better than the others. The mnemonics and rhymes by which we all learnt the various parts of the body might have changed, but the necessity of learning anatomy hasn't, nor is there any substitute to using a human corpse to learn from. Interestingly, new medical schools that have tried to teach anatomy using computers, textbooks and plastic models instead of corpses have had to revert to the old-fashioned methods: there really isn't a substitute for a three-dimensional understanding of the body's intricacy – and individuality – that we all learnt in the dissecting room from those bodies so generously willed to science. Similarly, learning about pathology and bacteriology brought to life textbook diagnoses and made sense of the causes of illness and their implications.

Looking back, perhaps there is another reason that Sir Andrew's approach to medicine resonated so strongly with me – why, if I was going to be a surgeon, I would want to model myself on him rather than on ones like the irascible Sir Lancelot Spratt – the surgeon played by James Robertson Justice in the *Doctor* series of films. Most medical students only get to see an operation in their fifth year. It would be strange if they did not identify most with the surgeon and his or her team. This, after all, is the practical purpose of so much of what they have spent the last four years cramming into their heads. But two years before I witnessed an operation as a medical student, I had already been allowed to watch one. And perhaps the circumstances might go a small way towards explaining why I identify so strongly with patients, and why patient-centred medicine is so important to me.

During the summer vacations in my first three years as a medical student, I worked at Stobhill Hospital in north Glasgow. In my last job there I was a theatre porter, collecting patients from their wards and taking them to the operating theatre. When the staff realised I was a medical student, they let me watch and told me what they were doing. I did hear of some Spratt-like behaviour from the surgeons, but not enough to make me want to change the direction of my career. Theatre porters see patients at their most fearful and vulnerable, or at least trying very hard to keep up their spirits. As you wheel them in through the swing doors towards the operating table, they are invariably worried and anxious, and you cannot help but hope that everything is going to work out well for them. Then your job is over, the staff there are starting to introduce themselves to your patient, and you go back to the wards. But you wouldn't be human if you didn't start thinking what the whole process looked like from the patient's point of view.

It all seems such a long time ago now, and of course it was. There weren't any disposable instruments back then, so all the needles and syringes had to be cleaned by hand before sterilising, and then checked to make sure they were sharp and had no rough edges. At Stobhill's Mental Health Unit, where I worked the previous year on a rehabilitation ward, they still used a coal fire to heat the ward. The unit was run efficiently but a lot more strictly than we have subsequently become used to. On one occasion, after taking a patient's temperature, I shook the thermometer to get the mercury down and accidentally broke it against the bed. This was a major incident. I had to pick up the pieces and place them in a kidney dish, covered with a clean towel, and go to matron and apologise, which I duly did. My wages were docked to pay for the damage.

Being a student wasn't all about studying. Sport was also important. At first, this meant rugby. I resumed my role as hooker and was playing in one game for the university when I almost broke my neck. I must have been paying attention in anatomy class, though, because as I was carried off, I was heard to shout: 'It's my greater occipital nerve!' I lost all feeling in my scalp for several weeks, and gave up playing serious rugby a little while later, realising quite sensibly that everyone else was much too big for me. I did, however, captain an occasional – and not very serious – team. The Mudlarks were, technically, the university's fifth xv, but team selection was quite random and usually consisted of whoever I could persuade to join me when I went to the Men's Union at lunch-time on Saturday with a few extra boots and jerseys. After this, I changed to hockey, which I really enjoyed. Or at least I did until one Saturday a hockey ball hit my toe, shot up under my chin and knocked out a few of my teeth. Miraculously, I found a dentist on Sunday and he pulled a few remnants from my gums. For me and hockey, however, it was the end of the line.

The Medico-Chirurgical Society was altogether less dangerous. It put on a series of events over the year and I volunteered to be its librarian. The library was housed in the Men's Union and in the Bridie Library, which was named after the playwright James Bridie.[3] The Bridie Library had a number of murals on the wall and the one I remember best goes:

> Open your window the night is beastly dark
> The phantoms are singing in the West End Park
> Open your window your love plain to see
> I'm here all alone, and there's nobody here but me.

I subsequently became the editor of *Surgo*, the society's journal, and eventually became president. To celebrate the centenary of Joseph Lister's first use antiseptic fluid – in this case, carbolic acid – to clean the wound of an 11-year-old boy – the university staged a major symposium. And as Lister had also been an honorary president of the Medico-Chirurgical Society, we held a centenary ball in his honour. Each year there was also a competition for the best student presentation and when, a few years later, I became the honorary president, I presented the society with a small trophy for the winner. It was put together by my brother from surgical instruments soldered onto an upturned kidney dish. I got to know my fellow students well in both my years and we decided we would hold reunions every five to ten years. These have indeed happened and it has been great to keep in touch with colleagues and friends and to see how well their careers have developed. We continue to meet but as we get older we have decided to meet every three years!

I was not particularly involved in student politics but regularly attended debates in the Union, dominated at the time by Donald Dewar (subsequently Scotland's inaugural First Minister) and John Smith, leader of the Labour Party who died suddenly in 1994, Jimmy Young (Lord Young of Strathblane) and Menzies Campbell (Lord Campbell of Pittenweem and now chancellor of St Andrews University). I also made friends with the legal philosopher Neil (subsequently Sir Neil) MacCormick, who persuaded me to join the Scottish National Party, which I duly did and have the membership card at home to prove it. Before his untimely death in 2009, we corresponded, and he recalled asking me to join. At the time we were both students, the SNP was committed to home rule, not independence, and that seemed appropriate for me. Many years later, when I chaired the Commission on Scottish Devolution, he sent me a copy of *A Flag in the Wind*, a book his father had published in 1955, which set out the history of the nationalist movement in Scotland and was important background reading. I also joined the Liberal Club, where Jo Grimond was the leader at the time and also a supporter of home rule.

As a medical student, I had just about enough money to run a car. My second-hand Ford Prefect was a long way from being in mint condition, and I seemed to be forever changing the spark plugs or altering the carburettor. It was never a good starter, especially in the cold weather, although I found that draining the water from the radiator at night, and filling it with hot water in the morning, made a real difference. One day, when my brother was driving it, the brakes failed and while he was trying to stop, he collided with a lamppost. From the bill Glasgow City Council then sent me, I can inform you that in 1966 a new lamp-post set you back £17 11s. All in all, we didn't have too much luck with the car, and before long it needed a new rear axle. With a few friends, including Roger Quinn, a future vascular surgeon, we took the car to a dump where another Prefect had been left. We lifted them up and changed the axles. Excellent training for aspiring surgeons!

Both Roger and I got through our degree and graduated on 6 July 1967. Two days after taking the Hippocratic Oath, I made another lifelong commitment when Ann and I got married. We had our honeymoon on Skye, and – this being a typical Scottish summer – the wind was so strong that it blew the windscreen wipers off our car. I also realised that I didn't have a coat and had to borrow my brother's. In spite of all that, we had a wonderful time. On Tuesday 1 August 1967, we were back in Glasgow. It was my first day as a junior doctor in Glasgow's Western Infirmary and my adventures in medicine were about to begin.

CHAPTER 3

A Surgeon in Training

OVER 250 YEARS AGO, qualifying as a surgeon was relatively easy. In his novel *Roderick Random* (1748), Tobias Smollett described the examination his eponymous hero had to pass in order to qualify as a naval surgeon. At the Royal College of Surgeons' Hall in London he was asked just five questions: could he explain how to trepan a patient; had he seen an amputation performed; how should one treat a florid patient injured in a fall; how should an intestinal wound be treated; and how would he behave if, while at sea, he was presented with a patient whose head had just been shot off. To the last question – perhaps a test of his equanimity – Random answered that he didn't know; he'd never seen such a thing. At the end of his three-year apprenticeship, though, that was all it took: five questions and a five-shilling fee – and young Roderick was free to work as a naval surgeon in George II's Britain.[1]

Though Smollett and I had our medical education in the same city, and at the same university, it took me rather longer and was a lot harder. Getting a degree in medicine was only half the battle. Without full registration from the General Medical Council, no-one is allowed to practise medicine, and for that I had to spend a year as a resident house officer at Glasgow's Western Infirmary. In the medical hierarchy, house officers were the lowest of the low. Their duties were confined to the basics: clerking patients in when they arrived, making sure all the investigations requested were performed, checking that blood was cross-matched and that patients were comfortable after their operation, looking after them until they were ready to be discharged, and so on. All of this was a satisfying process, even if somewhat routine. The hours were long – 20-hour days were not uncommon – and when I did finally get to doze off in my bed next to the ward office, sleep was invariably interrupted by a request to attend to a patient. I was living, sleeping and dreaming my job, and occasionally the dividing line between those states of being disappeared. I can still remember the surprised looks I got when I turned up at A&E one night at four in the morning. I wasn't actually on the rota, nor was there any emergency. I must just have dreamed that there was.

Ann and I bought a second top floor flat in Rupert Street, just off the Great Western Road as it reaches St George's Cross, although because of my job I spent far less time there than I would have wished. As we had very little money, an uncle who owned a lorry helped us by driving round our relatives picking up chairs and tables and assorted bits of furniture they no longer needed. The flat had a large and long hall, which was great for parties, when it was used for bowls, darts and other games.

At this stage, I was thinking of specialising as a dermatologist. That, after all, was what the PhD thesis I was still trying to finish was all about and, had Sir Andrew Kay not asked me to join his surgery unit at the Western the following year and train as a senior house officer, that is almost certainly what I would have become. Given my admiration for him, though, that was an offer I couldn't refuse. So in 1968, for the princely salary of £1,470 per year, I became Hall Fellow in Surgery. I was taught by the very best. That year, I worked with Tom Gibson, one of the finest plastic surgeons in the country. During the Second World War, he had worked at the Burns Unit in Glasgow Royal Infirmary, where his pioneering 1943 paper on skin grafts has been hailed as 'the work which first placed the laws of transplantation on a firm scientific basis'. When Sir Peter Medawar, his co-author on that paper, won the Nobel Prize in 1960 for his work on immunological tolerance, he acknowledged that its roots lay in the research he and Gibson had done together in Glasgow. I worked with Gibson at the Canniesburn Plastic Surgery and Burns Unit. He was so skilled, and it was wonderful to watch him perform operations. I learned so much from him about delicacy of touch and attention to detail. He also had a talent for writing light-hearted verse about his colleagues and profession, and that was something I have tried to do too.

Having mentors such as Kay and Gibson confirmed me in my wish to become a surgeon, but the rest of the team were hardly any less impressive. If a measure of the regard in which a surgical team is held is the extent to which its members are headhunted by other hospitals and institutions, then the teaching of surgery at the Western in Glasgow was in the middle of a golden age.[2] Of course, what we could do as surgeons back then was far more limited than it is now, just as some of the operations we had to perform then are now hardly ever needed. On Mondays, for example, we used to have a full-day peptic ulcer clinic, in which pre- and post-operative patients were seen and surgical management discussed. Ten years later, and thanks to groundbreaking research on peptic ulceration, this surgery was replaced by antibacterial treatment. Another difference between then and now is that hospitals tended not to have any formally designated Intensive Care Unit, although at the Western Professor Iain Ledingham had established one in the surgery unit for what he called his 'shock team'. His own particular interest was in hyperbaric medicine and he was examining the use of high-pressure chambers in the management of illness – another fruitful line of research.

All this time my skills as a surgeon were improving. I passed my primary exams to be a Fellow of the Royal College of Surgeons (Glasgow) in 1968, and was working hard towards taking the final FRCS exams. As part of a busy surgical unit there was a fair share of acute surgical practice, and this again was invaluable experience. Having to make quick decisions and to act rapidly, often in the face of incomplete information, was a real lesson in responsibility. Again, it fitted in well with my future role as Chief Medical Officer.

Another skill I was learning was how to impart information crisply and clearly. This was something I picked up while rehearsing the presentation of papers at scientific meetings within the Department of Surgery. At these meetings, the staff tended not to hold back if they had any criticism, which further underlined the importance of thorough preparation. As criticism often centred on the slides used (this was, remember, in the distant days before PowerPoint) I valued the advice of Gabriel Donald, the head of the Medical Illustrations Department, who helped with their creation. After I left the department I always pre-presented all such papers to Ann for her comments.

As well as studying hard for my exams, I had also been writing papers of my own. Interestingly, given the direction my career was about to turn, one of the first I published while in the surgical unit was about the information sent to GPs revealing precisely what cancer patients had been told about their illness while in hospital. The answer, it turned out, was hardly anything. After looking at heaps of letters from the unit to GPs, I discovered that while there was plenty of information about the operation, including the kind of stitches used, few letters mentioned what the patient had been told about their illness or even whether they had been given the diagnosis in the first place. This, I hasten to remind you, was in the early 1970s, we have come a long way since then.

In 1970, I was awarded a PhD for my dermatology thesis and – the two weren't linked – appointed lecturer in surgery at the Western Infirmary. I also began writing books. I have had a particularly varied career, and in hindsight, seem to have marked each change of direction by writing about the job I've just finished. *Basic Skills for the Surgical Housemen* was the first of these.[3] It came out in 1971, the same year I passed my FRCS examination – easily the hardest exams I have ever taken. I was a surgeon at last. But what kind of surgeon? What was going to be my specialism? And would it be something I would commit to for life, building up an expertise year by year – or would I want to stay true to my inner philomath and be lured away by some other subject?

In the early 1970s transplantation was the cutting edge of medical research, and I was becoming increasingly fascinated by it. This was largely due to my immediate boss, Mr Peter Bell, who was just back from Denver, where he had been working with Thomas Starzl (1926–2017), the American surgeon who had performed the world's first successful liver transplant in 1967 at the University of Colorado Health Sciences Center. Thanks to what he learnt in the US, Peter – now Professor Sir Peter, to give him his correct title – got Glasgow's transplantation programme up and running before he left to take up the inaugural surgery chair at Leicester. A genial Yorkshireman with a great sense of humour, I was particularly sorry to see him go. Before he did, though, he taught me how best to connect patients to dialysis machines and together Peter and I published a book on the subject.[4]

He was one of my great mentors and great fun to work with.

I was already interested in transplantation, as it linked in neatly with my work on the MD research degree on organ preservation that I began straight after finishing my PhD. My research involved perfusing rats' hearts to preserve them and seeing how long we could keep them viable for re-transplantation. These days, I am more conscious of the broader issues of the use of animals in research. Ethics became a focus of interest later in my career. During this time, my first two children, Andrew and Lynn, were born, in 1970 and 1971 respectively, and we moved to Earlbank Avenue, an end-terrace three-bedroomed house in Scotstoun. Bart, our first flatcoat retriever, soon joined us. We moved churches too, from Lansdowne to Scotstoun East, and I became a Church of Scotland elder in both. In 1971, I applied for, and was awarded, a Medical Research Council fellowship for a year's research (1972–1973). As immunology was at the basis of much of the new research into more effective transplants, I went to the Chester Beatty Research Institute, part of the Royal Marsden Hospital in London, to study it under Professor Tony Davies and his team.

The following year, a few days before I took up the new job, we travelled down to London. We took the overnight sleeper with the car and arrived safely in London at Kensington Olympia – but when we got the car off the train, there was no sign of Bart. He had, it turned out, been sent on the boat train to Paris. Somehow we managed to contact the train and Bart was returned to Victoria station, where I was told to pick him up. When I tried to do this, the officials clearly thought that I was pulling a fast one. Bart, they were convinced, must have come in from France and I was obviously trying to evade British quarantine restrictions. I did my best to convince them, but they still didn't believe me. Only when I told them that I was a surgeon and wouldn't dream of taking such health risks did they finally relent and allow me to be reunited with Bart.[5]

We rented a house in Wimbledon where Andrew attended the local nursery and soon started speaking in a marked south London accent which took some time to reverse when we returned to Scotland. On the plus side, both he and Lynn were very taken with the Wombles of Wimbledon Common, whose TV series began while we were living nearby, and they loved going out to look for them. This was the first

time we had lived outside Glasgow and – at the risk of sounding he-
retical – the Dear Green Place seemed dull by comparison. Much as
I loved it, Byres Road just had that little bit less going on than King's
Road, Chelsea, which was just around the corner from us at the Chester Beatty Research Institute. And for me, at least, the work going on
inside the institute was even more exciting.

My research project was to try to find out why there were fewer
tumours in the small bowel than in the large bowel. Was there an
immunological reason? Was it just because the food passed through
more quickly? Or was there another reason altogether? The staff in
the group were all very helpful, and I still keep in touch with Bob Ker-
bel, now long back in Canada. We got on very well, not least because
I was taller than he was! The regular weekly seminars introduced me
to new ideas, and I met a fascinating range of people. I attended a
few clinics at the Royal Marsden to get a feel for the kind of work
they were doing and to meet the senior medical staff. These days it is
hard to imagine, but back then medical oncology was in its infancy,
and Britain's two centres of excellence in cancer treatment – St Bart-
holomew's Hospital (Bart's) and the Royal Marsden – were both in
London. The people I got to know there were deeply impressive. Gordon Hamilton Fairley, the Australian who was Britain's first professor
of medical oncology, was particularly so: an expert in immunology, he
was hard at work trying to find more effective forms of chemotherapy
when he was killed by an IRA bomb in 1975. New Zealand-born Tim
McElwain, his protégé, who had just been appointed senior lecturer at the Royal Marsden when I arrived, was already developing a
stellar reputation for his work in modifying chemotherapy treatments
for patients with Hodgkin's disease, vastly improving their chances of
survival.

But one of the most important people I met at the Royal Marsden
was someone whose work wasn't so much part of the fight against
cancer as the fight against the suffering of the terminally ill. By 1972,
when I first met Cicely Saunders, the first hospice she built – St Christopher's, in Sydenham – had already been open for five years. In his
new biography of Cicely, my Glasgow university colleague, David
Clark, shows quite brilliantly how she revolutionised care for the terminally ill, who had been all but neglected in the first quarter-century

of the NHS.[6] St Christopher's was a showcase of what was possible, and I soon became a regular visitor. There had been hospices before, of course, often places founded at the start of the last century by religious orders. They were places where the terminally ill could often receive good nursing and spiritual care but where there wasn't any sustained attempt to relieve physical suffering. This, Saunders realised, was an appalling failure of care. Decades of thought and experience in looking after dying patients as a nurse, social worker, and, finally, as a trained doctor, had taught her that a new kind of hospice was needed – one in which a specialised, multidisciplinary team could concentrate on offering the dying relief from both pain and mental stress, as well as doing their best to offer consolation to the bereaved.

The first patients at St Christopher's were mainly – though not exclusively – suffering from cancer. For many people at the time, cancer was the C-word, a taboo unmentionable except in worried, whispered conversations, so in taking on one late 20th century taboo subject – death – Cicely was also, at least partially, taking on another. She was also doing so in a way that defied some of the more bureaucratic conventions of the time. One woman who was subsequently to play an important role in the hospice movement explained that the reason she first became interested in it was when she met the wife of a neighbour who had been admitted to St Christopher's from a hospital. The first thing they had done was to cut the hospital number tags from his wrist. 'You're not a number, you're a person,' they told him. Or, in Saunders' words, quoted on her hospice's website to this day:

> You matter because you are you. You matter to the last moment
> of your life, and we will do all we can to help you not only to die
> peacefully, but also to live until you die.

In the early 1970s, patient-centred care along these lines was still in its infancy. So too was the idea of a team-centred approach. Yet at the Royal Marsden, this was already a reality and I had seen for myself how senior surgeon Ronald Raven insisted on collaboration between radiotherapists, chemotherapists, and pathologists to plan the best possible result for his cancer patients. Before too long, I would find myself putting that lesson into practice too, and as I was also influenced by Raven's work on the rehabilitation and continuing care of cancer patients, I am doubly indebted to him.

Yet it's Saunders who casts an even longer shadow of influence on my life. I think the reason is that although it's patently untrue to say that until she came along all terminally ill patients died neglected and in pain, it *is* true to say that no-one did more than her to lessen the odds of that happening. The palliative care revolution she had introduced at St Christopher's – one in which, thanks to her, Britain led the world – was already underway during my time in London. In November 1972, for example, the first national symposium was held there, its proceedings written up in the *British Medical Journal*. The following year Richard Lamerton – whom I also soon got to know – published his book *Care for the Dying*. Recognition of palliative care by the Royal College of Physicians as a medical specialism in its own right was still a full 15 years away, but the subject was already pulling away from the margins.

As ever in medicine, a revolution in care isn't just the work of one person – even one as forceful, charismatic and committed as Cicely Saunders. I have been privileged enough to get to know many of those whose work ensured that the palliative care revolution took hold – people like Robert Twycross, who did such great work comparing the efficacy of morphine or diamorphine in palliative care, or Colin Murray Parkes, who set up St Christopher's bereavement service and went on to become one of the world's great experts in the subject. Many others had joined them in the great cause of cementing its place as a core specialism, and in 2012, I had the privilege of chairing a witness seminar, organised by the Wellcome Trust, on the subject of 'Palliative Care in the UK 1970–2010' which several of them attended.

By 2012 it was 40 years since I first met Dame (as she subsequently became) Cicely. Four whole decades since I first was shown round St Christopher's and caught a glimpse of what the future of end-of-life care could be. Forty years on, in both the Alan Bennett play and the Harrow school song of that name, such a passage of time is an occasion for elegiac memories, but in this case this reunion of colleagues was a cause for pride, not sadness. The hospice revolution the attendees at the seminar had all brought about hadn't always been plain sailing: there had been tensions between public and privately funded hospices, uncertainties over the extent to which they should be faith-based, whether they were to be specialist units or 'homes from home'. At the start, hospices had even been treated with a degree of suspicion: 'Abandon hope all ye who enter here' was the headline over the newspaper story about the opening of a hospice in Sheffield in 1971.[7] It took time for such attitudes to shift, and for nicknames like 'Dr Death' for hospice doctors to vanish into history. Yet the attendees at the seminar – or at least those with a 40-year rearview mirror – had seen that happen, and they could look back with a fair degree of satisfaction. They had helped make medical history – and, more importantly, had helped take some pain out of the world, which is the reason most of us go into medicine in the first place.

All of this, though, is to zoom four decades into the future. Back in 1973, my research year in London had finished and I was back working in Glasgow as a surgeon. I was looking to move up the career ladder. Though I say it myself, I was a strong candidate: just 32, but already qualified as a surgeon with two doctorates, a science degree, scores of papers and a Surgical Research Society Prize to my name. If anyone had been looking for a surgeon with a special interest in vascular and transplant surgery, I would have been their man, but there were no such jobs. Week in, week out, I scanned the *BMJ*, looking for a job like that. Week in, week out, there wasn't one. And then one day that summer, I got a phone call. There *was* a job I might be interested in, I was told. It was a higher grade than I had even thought about applying for, and it was in Glasgow, so I wouldn't have to move. True, it was in a field of medicine I'd never previously thought about working in, and because I would be starting an entire project from scratch, it would almost certainly be a very challenging job. Would I at least consider it?

CHAPTER 4

Scotland's First Oncology Unit

'PROFESSOR TO LEAD research into cancer' said the headline in *The Scotsman* on 28 August 1974, and if you read that you might have assumed that the person appointed Glasgow University's – indeed, Scotland's – first professor of oncology to head a £500,000 project was already a trained oncologist of sorts. And I wasn't. You might, too, have assumed that premises for the project had already been acquired and perhaps some of the staff too, because the Cancer Research Campaign's statement went on to promise that the new department of oncology would be staffed by academically trained clinicians who were 'broadly based in experience and outward-looking in attitude'. But while that would happen, it hadn't yet.

The newspaper had, however, got one thing right. This was news: there was nothing like the university's new department anywhere else in Scotland. It was a huge and significant project, but it was starting from scratch. The department, at that stage, didn't exist at all: no building, no staff, no beds, no patients, no office, no telephone, not even a typewriter. So how, you might reasonably wonder, did I get the job in the first place? Well, I must admit, it wouldn't happen now. But back then, oncology was only just becoming established as a specialism in its own right.[1] Of the few oncologists there were, in places like the Royal Marsden and Bart's, the prospect of leaving such havens of cutting-edge research for an institution where they would have to assemble their own team, search out their own premises, fund-raise for future projects and generally find their own professional way in a new city, clearly didn't appeal.

Because I had just come back to Glasgow from the Chester Beatty, and knew many potential candidates in London, I was asked whom

I would recommend for the professorship. I suggested a number of people whom I thought would do an excellent job and left it at that. Until I got that phone call suggesting that I apply myself I hadn't even thought of doing so. Forty years later, talking to a distinguished surgeon, Professor Stuart MacPherson, with whom I had worked in Glasgow, I found out what had been going on behind the scenes. He had been at the American College of Surgeons' meeting in Chicago in 1973, where he met Sir Andrew Kay, who invited him to dinner. They had discussed Glasgow's new chair of oncology and the difficulties they were having in filling the position. The reason for the difficulty was that the job had two key requirements. They needed a clinician, but because research and the link-up with the university were key parts of the Cancer Research Campaign's brief, that clinician needed to be somebody with a science degree and a background in the kind of research I had just finished at the Chester Beatty. The problem with filling the job was that a lot of the eminently qualified scientists didn't have a clinical background and many of the clinicians lacked a strong training in science.

'I wonder,' said Sir Andrew, 'do you think wee Kenny could be the person to do it?' My friend agreed that wee Kenny probably could.

So that's how it was that in October 1974, Professor KC Calman turned up for work at his alma mater. At 32, I may well have been the youngest professor on the university's entire staff, and the professorship gave me the rank of consultant too. Such a sudden climb up the career ladder, missing out a couple of rungs on the way, caused a certain amount of resentment among those who had been forced to wait until their 50s before attaining such heady heights. To make things worse, I was a very young-looking 32. Just how young-looking was brought home to me one lunchtime when I was queuing up in the hospital's dining room. There were always two queues – one for junior staff and a generally shorter one for consultants and professors. When I joined this queue, the staff refused to serve me because I looked too young for my job. In the end, a distinguished cardiologist had to come to my rescue. 'He really is a professor, you know,' the unconvinced lady with the ladle was told, but she let me through.

Already, thanks in part to what I had learnt from Cicely Saunders at St Christopher's, my interest in cancer extended to the total care of the patient 'including the social, psychological and interpersonal relationships which are so crucial': that at least was also spelt out in *The Scotsman*'s story. But I had to do a lot more than that too. The news story had mentioned that we would be concentrating on the cancers of the gastrointestinal tract, breast and lung which together accounted for 60 per cent of all cancers in Scotland. As a surgeon, I had already had some experience of operating on the more common cancers, but now I would no longer be doing any of that. Instead of using my surgeon's scalpel, I would be a physician trying to provide cancer patients with the best medication, best standards of care, and best possible outcomes, and leading a research team in a variety of projects that would allow us to do all of that even more effectively.

I was under no illusions about the importance of the job. The Cancer Research Campaign wanted to build up a network of five specialised cancer centres by 1983. Manchester was the first to be established, and Glasgow was the second, chosen ahead of anywhere else in Scotland for two key reasons: first, the high-quality research into cancer already going on at the Beatson Institute and secondly because, with 2.5 million people in the newly-formed Strathclyde region alone, the size of the population warranted it. Historically, Glasgow had often been in the forefront of cancer care. In 1890, the ten-bed hospital at 163 Hill Street was one of the world's first to be dedicated entirely to the disease and six years later, the man who ran it, Dr (later Sir) George Beatson – after whom the Beatson Institute is named – pioneered a key operation that is still occasionally used in the treatment of breast cancer. Two years before the outbreak of the First World War, that hospital, by now renamed the Royal Glasgow Cancer Hospital, was one of the first in the world to have its own cancer research department. There was a lot to live up to.

My first year, however, was difficult. Although I had an excellent secretary (Marion McLeod), we didn't have a proper office – just a room in the nurses' home in the Western Infirmary. It was so basic that it didn't even have modern power points, so we had to rely on an extended cable to use our new electronic typewriter. I could at least start assembling the team, and with Gordon McVie as senior lecturer and Mike Soukup as senior registrar, we had some of the best in the cancer-fighting business, as they both went on to prove in their subsequent careers.[2] Dr Stan Kaye then joined us and was an enormous help to me.

What we didn't have were patients – or at least ones who weren't already beyond treatment. In the first six months of our existence, 60 per cent of patients died in a month without treatment for their cancer. That one statistic was a challenge to everything I wanted the new department of oncology to be. Of course we wanted to provide care near the end of life, but that wasn't our main purpose. We wanted to be able to bring hope, to harness the very best available research and use it to extend lives, to make sure that our patients had the best chance of fighting their cancer, and to learn from them as they did so. Palliative care was part of our job, but only part. Our ambitions, our optimism, our energy, our morale, maybe even our commitment to research might begin to crumble if we were denied the opportunity to make a difference.

Why, I wondered, were the only patients being referred to us so often ones who were already almost beyond help? Why were we hardly being sent any who could benefit from the new treatments we could introduce? The answer, I came to realise, reflected a suspicion of new specialisms that is probably par for the course in the history of medicine. Medical oncology – researching, diagnosing, treating and managing cancer – had only been officially accredited as a speciality three years previously. Some surgeons, especially those who didn't realise the potential of the new anti-cancer drugs, genuinely didn't understand what we could do. After all, they routinely removed tumours as part of their general surgical duties, as I had done myself. Surely they couldn't think that the new treatments were some kind of implicit criticism of their work? So what was the reason?

One day, I was talking this through with a distinguished professor of orthopaedics, who had moved to Glasgow in 1942 as the university's first lecturer in the subject and set up a similar kind of department (involving both academic research and treatment) to the one I was trying to establish in medical oncology.[3] At the time, orthopaedics didn't exist as a separate specialism, and was handled by general surgeons. In the first year that his department was up and running, he told me, they only gave him their worst cases – for example, bones with multiple fractures and oozing pus. 'See what you can do with that, then, professor,' they'd tell him. I recognised the parallel immediately. But the lesson I took away from the encounter was a positive one. After all, the department my colleague had set up had gone on to achieve an international reputation. So, I determined, with enthusiasm, good relations with colleagues in other disciplines, teamwork, and above all by proven results, would ours.

By 1975 we had our own laboratories and had started fundraising for our research projects. I had also established a good working relationship with the head of the Beatson Institute, Professor John Paul, and the two of us together wrote a short medical primer on cancer.[4] Dr Ian Freshney joined the team from the Beatson at a time when it was developing a wider range of interests and our research base extended even further. Gradually, as medical oncology became established, any residual suspicion of our work dissolved and more and more patients were referred to us. From this we began a wide range of clinical groups involving clinicians from across the West of Scotland. These were generally chaired by staff from outside of the Department, and there were strong links with radiotherapy and haematology. Clinical trials were established and there were regular meetings to feedback information.

Right from the start, I had determined that we would learn from the best oncologists in the world. The first to visit us was Lucien Israel, a French oncologist with a wealth of experience both in America and Europe, where he had chaired the Brussels-based European Organisation for Research into Treatment of Cancers.[5] We learnt much from him, not only about the range of new treatments available but about the importance of taking the patient along with the research and making sure of consent and comprehension at every stage. From the Vincent T Lombardi Cancer Center and the US National Cancer Institute – still flush with funds from the 'war on cancer' Nixon had declared back in 1971 – came Philip Schein, who put us in touch with latest developments in drug research. Paul Carbone, whose researches into combination chemotherapy had already greatly extended the lives of those with advanced Hodgkin's disease, involved us in the multi-centre clinical trial group he ran at the University of Wisconsin in Madison.[6] Joining this placed Glasgow patients right at the leading edge of research in cancer treatment and prevention.

In the 1970s, such trials and treatments were being introduced all the time, and it was important to be fully aware of what they could do for our patients and what, if they agreed to participate in clinical trials, our patients could do for them. As oncologists, we well knew how wide of the mark all those newspaper stories about miracle breakthroughs would turn out to be, how long the process of testing would take before accreditation, and how many false dawns there would invariably be before that happened. But we knew too that the way in which ordinary people talked about cancer – or more accurately, didn't talk about cancer – was wrong. Because it really wasn't the lost cause of popular imagination, the hopeless and inevitable end that relatives had in mind when they begged nurses not to tell loved ones that they had cancer. There was hope, but it was almost impossible to quantify, and it grew in the most unlikely places.

Let me give you one example. It's the story of the discovery of a drug called cisplatin and it is a favourite of mine because it proves the value – measurable, if it is not too melodramatic to point out, in human lives – of pure science.[7] I knew some of the people who played a major role in its introduction, and it overlaps my career as a clinician rather neatly. If I think fondly about cisplatin, it is because it is one of those treatments whose introduction in the late '70s I witnessed bringing new hope where there was little, if any, before.

The story starts in a lab in East Lansing, Michigan in 1965. Barnett Rosenberg, a biophysics professor, and a microbiologist called Loretta van Camp, were trying to find out what happened when they ran an electric current through some E.coli bacteria. And what happened was very interesting indeed, because as soon as the electrodes were put into the bacteria, it started to form long strands. This, they gradually realised, was nothing to do with the electricity and everything to do with the platinum electrodes. The multi-million-dollar question was obvious: if platinum could inhibit cell division in fast-growing bacteria, would it do the same thing for cancer cells?

Fears about toxicity meant that the Americans didn't push ahead with research into precisely which of the platinum-based compounds Rosenberg had identified as having the potential to kill cancer cells would do so most efficiently. But Sir Alexander Haddow, then head of the Chester Beatty Research Institute, realised the significance of

Rosenberg's discoveries and put a pharmacologist called Dr Tom Connors on the case. Connors – whom I got to know when I worked at the Chester Beatty – worked out that of all the various platinum compounds, the most likely candidate to work well and safely was Cisplatin [$PtCl_2(NH_3)_2$].

This was in 1971, the year before I started work at the Chester Beatty on my own project. At the Royal Marsden, Dr Eve Wiltshaw began clinical trials of cisplatin with a group of 20 women suffering from ovarian cancer. At a conference in Oxford the following year, she was able to report encouraging results – even though all of her patients had been seriously ill and had already undergone radiotherapy. An American cancer researcher reported finding similar benefits while treating testicular cancers in a paper published in 1974. Four years later, cisplatin was approved by the US Food and Drug administration and went into general use on both sides of the Atlantic.

Meanwhile in Glasgow, by 1978 we had already moved to a new hospital. At Gartnavel General, a mile and a half away to the north-west of the university, we finally had our own ward, a dedicated space for ten patients and their families. Space was limited and the hospital authorities built a small office next to the lifts for administrative staff – who then refused to use it. I took it over as my office and Ann made some curtains to make it more private. Ward 7B was nine floors above the ground, with a great view over the city. When I think of all the places I have worked in, my memory circles back to those beds, the patients I met there and the staff I worked with. There's nothing there for me now – in fact, I don't even know whether the ward is in use – and yet it remains hugely important to me. I still remember giving cisplatin to my first patient there in 1978. In my time in the department at the Western, no-one with testicular cancer had ever been referred to us. There would have been no point. The only possible treatment was surgery, and at medical oncology we were on a different path. A path that, until now, had not been open, even though testicular cancer was, and is, the most common cancer in young men.

Cisplatin made such a difference to what we could do. Before too long, the death rate from testicular cancer had completely fallen away from what it was in 1971; or to put it another way, now more than 80 per cent of our patients could expect to be cured. There was a risk of infertility, and we had to set up ways of storing the patient's sperm as a precaution – although these days fertility usually recovers within two or three years. There were, of course, setbacks too. Cisplatin wasn't everything we hoped it would be. It might save lives, but it could often leave long-term damage on the kidneys, nerves and hearing. It also induced vomiting in every single patient on every single occasion they took it. Because patients always associated it with me, they would even be sick as soon as they saw me. You get used to it.

But science doesn't stay still. If cisplatin always induced vomiting, how could we make drugs that wouldn't have that effect? And as we came to understand the precise chemical mechanisms by which cisplatin worked – how it bound itself to DNA and killed off cancer cells – couldn't we retain its functionality while reducing its toxicity? When I went down to the Chester Beatty in 1971, its head of applied chemistry was an extrovert Londoner called Ken Harrap. In 1976, with the help of chemists at Johnson Matthey, he started work on what was to become carboplatin, a revised molecular reboot of cisplatin without its harmful effects. Licensed in the UK in 1986, it then went on to be one of the world's best-selling anti-cancer drugs.

I mention people like Ken, or Tom Connors, or Eve Wiltshaw not because I knew them especially well but because their story was, for the time I was a medical oncologist, mine too. When I look back, though, I can't help but see the legacy they left behind and on which medicine is continuing to build. They, and their whole generation of cancer researchers, deserve to be celebrated. They were pioneers, opening up vast prairies of research, and the intellectual excitement about the discoveries they made carried us all through the long hours we worked, whether in the lab or on the wards. We could read the journals and see tantalising signs of progress almost everywhere. This was the decade in which combination chemotherapy was first coming into widespread use, when for the first time we could offer more than just surgery and radiotherapy, and actually turn back cancers which had spread.

In the late 1970s we set up a course on Basic Principles of Cancer Chemotherapy with Professor John Smyth from Edinburgh, and Professor Martin Tattersall from the University of Sydney. Professor JMA Whitehouse from Southampton was also involved. It brought lots of people together and we learned much from each, producing a book with the same title in 1980.[8] Our department reflected this cautiously growing optimism. The clinical trials we were running expanded and developed and became an important force for change, involving clinical units from across the whole of the West of Scotland. In 1983, for example, almost ten years after I set up the department, there were trials on breast cancer, advanced melanoma, gastric cancer, colon cancer, ovarian cancer, testicular teratomas, as well as work on new drug development. Each of these involved collaboration and leadership outwith the department. The clinical trials unit we set up was central to this.

Our research groups grew too. We were always concerned about weight loss during treatment and we set up one such group on nutrition and metabolism. Others looked into drug resistance to different types of tumours and a tumour biology group studying how cancer cells developed, while Professor Sandy Florence of Strathclyde University led a group looking at how cytotoxic drugs (ones which killed living cells) worked within the body. We were also accredited as the World Health Organisation Colon Cancer Centre, linking up with the West of Scotland Cancer Surveillance Unit as a focal point for epidemiological research studies into the disease, co-ordinating data on treatment, outcomes and pre-existing genetic information, in an attempt to also find out to what extent Scotland's high incidence of bowel cancer was directly related to the starchy food in the typical Scottish diet. This Cancer Surveillance Unit was led by Dr Charles Gillis, who provided the essential data managing background and encouraged this type of research. He was an inspiration to others, including Peter Boyle, who went on to great things in a European context. As the work developed, I regularly visited the Veterinary School at the University to meet Dr Andrew Nash, and we did a cancer clinic together. I learned a lot, and I hope some animals' health improved as a result of therapy. I also did clinics in Ayrshire at Ballochmyle Hospital and in Greenock.

One of the most important aspects of my work in the cancer unit was to build an effective team. Having social events, like our Christmas pantomime, helped: it was a good opportunity for staff to say what they really thought about their professor. I recall one special event when Dr Sam Ahmedzai, later to become a distinguished leader in palliative care, took the lead and sang a wonderful song about being an oncologist. The other thing I introduced was the Golden Pisspot award, given to the doctor whose research work most disrupted clinical care. I had painted a male pisspot gold and set it on a wooden bread board, and it was signed by the offender. When I left the department it was presented to me, signed by all staff, and still sits in my home. One of the things I have always done is to present gold stars to those who have done well, a great way of recognising special effort. I have continued to do this to special people including Ministers in Whitehall, distinguished scientists, and I always keep a few in my pocket. You never know how useful they might be!

In ten years we had done a lot. From a standing start, we had created a department with an international reputation and won funding for many important research projects. The staff we trained went on to make major contributions to cancer care, both nationally and internationally, and seeing them flourish has been a huge satisfaction. I am enormously proud of all of them. I am proud too to have known and worked with some of the scientists I have written about in this chapter, who made the first great strides in the new field of medical oncology. Yet when I look back at my time on Ward 7B, I also look back at the patients I met there with just as much gratitude. There are two reasons for that. First, because they too were very much part of that same medical revolution, and secondly, because they provided me with the greatest learning experience of my life. Those ten years were significant too because my children grew up. Throughout those years I used to wake them up each morning with a joke from a little joke book I had and they would throw things at me but at least they got up. It was great to watch them busy at school, Boys' Brigade, Brownies and Guides events. Andrew was into sport, rugby football and golf. Lynn played the flute and it was she who enjoyed dancing classes! As Susan grew up she enjoyed speaking at debates and meetings and these became one of her great interests. She also attended the Scottish Youth Theatre and played hockey.

CHAPTER 5

Learning from Patients

THE ROAD FROM Entebbe to Kampala runs across the top of a lake as big as Scotland. Drive seven miles along it, and you come to a tropical rainforest that edges down to a papyrus swamp which in turn marks the Ugandan shoreline on Lake Victoria. These days, much of the northern shore of the lake has been lost to ribbon development, but you can still see the tropical forest where, in 1947, Alexander Haddow came to research yellow fever but ended up discovering a new virus altogether. He named it after the place where he had made the discovery – a forest at the time known only to locals but now a name known to half the world. It would, he ordained, henceforth be known as the Zika virus.

We had many fascinating patients on Ward 7B but, to me at least, none quite like Alexander John Haddow – entomologist, virologist, epidemiologist, pibroch virtuoso, fellow-professor at the University of Glasgow, and friend. He came to us in 1977, and died the following year. If you had to sum him up in a sentence, you'd mention his groundbreaking work on the epidemiology of Burkitt's lymphoma, or the arboviruses (viruses transmitted by arthropods) he'd discovered, or his work transforming the research institute he worked at in Entebbe from 1942 to 1965 (the last 12 years as director) into the best of its kind in the world. After that, he returned to Glasgow University, where he had taken degrees in zoology and medicine and later worked as Dean of the Faculty of Medicine and Professor of Administrative Medicine. That, though, wouldn't convey the measure of the man. CVs – even of illustrious men – never do. You'd have to look deeper – to imagine, for example, what it must have been like working with him on the tower he built 75ft up into and above the canopy of the Zika tropical forest to catch mosquitoes. In order to find out more about how mosquitoes carry yellow fever, he insisted that they be collected from all six levels of the tower – the Haddow Tower, as it became known – and at all hours of the day and night. Here's how a friend of his described what happened as night fell atop the Haddow Tower in Zika forest:

> The everyday noises cease and are replaced by the eerie calls of the tree frogs or the croaks of bull frogs from a nearby swamp, the churring voice of nightjars or the hoot of owls, the shrill chirping of cicadas and the hum of the nocturnal mosquitoes. Dead silence is rare and is usually the presage of wind or rain, unappreciated by us but apparent to the more acute senses of the lower animals. The temperature drops and the humidity rises. We are kept busy dealing with the catch, in my own case, of anaesthetised monkeys which had to be kept warm with hot water bottles, for without the heat the mosquitoes would not be attracted. By about 3 or 4 o'clock in the morning, everyone longs for daybreak.[1]

Now, obviously most patients in Ward 7B would not have such esoteric memories. Most would not have made such (as it transpired nearly 70 years later, when we finally realised the full scale of the threat the Zika virus posed to humans) devastating discoveries, and most were not already friends. But that didn't lessen their individuality or importance: just as people are more than their CVs, they are more than their diagnoses too. We wanted to somehow express that in a symbol, a work of art that would spell out a commitment to a kind of care that was deeper and wider than the merely medical. And Alexander Haddow helped us to do just that.

He was, along with all his other prodigious skills, a quite remarkable artist – indeed, when, a couple of years ago, Glasgow University put together an exhibition based on the archive he had bequeathed to it, the detail and accuracy of his drawings of African wildlife was much commented on. Anyone who has seen the sketch he did, aged just seven, of a Yellow Fever-carrying mosquito (he was one of those people who knew from an early age what he wanted to be) wouldn't have been too surprised by that. But he was also, towards the end of his life, fascinated by Celtic art. This, he decided, would be the basis of the symbol he would provide for our oncology department. Traditionally in Celtic art, the triquentrum, or interlinked three-pointed knot, was used to symbolise the Trinity. If we made it a four-pointed knot, Alexander reasoned, it could stand as a symbol for all four methods of cancer treatment – surgery, radiotherapy, chemotherapy and immunotherapy – that were then potentially available. But because he realised that there was more to each of us than that, the four-pointed interlinked knot would have another level of symbolism. It would represent the four aspects of the patient: physical, psychological, emotional and spiritual. All four of the leaves would be bound together by a circle, a giant 'O' threading unbreakably over and under each of them. This would represent the Department of Oncology, which would – symbolically at least – also hold those two levels of meaning together.

But what would all of those ambitions we had for the department actually mean in practice? How could we make them real, and not just a vague aspiration or well-meaning waffle? What did we have to do to look after our patients' psychological, emotional and spiritual needs? In years to come, 'patient-centred care' would become – quite rightly – an NHS mantra.[2] In the 1970s, it wasn't – although in hindsight what we were doing on Ward 7B was edging towards it. Already we had made some changes to the way in which the department was run. Rather than having our patients needlessly waiting, we adopted a 'team approach' in which the work of the nursing staff, dieticians, physiotherapists, pharmacists, pathologists and psychologists was integrated. Let me give an example of how this worked. Before the major clinics, when we saw 30–40 patients in a morning, the team had a preparatory meeting attended by doctors, nurses, a pharmacist, a dietician, and a psychologist. As we went through each patient on the list, we checked their needs and wrote down who should see the patient first. For example, some patients might be having trouble with their drugs, and the pharmacist might be best to begin the consultation. Another would involve the dietician. Those who might require chemotherapy that morning needed a blood check first, and this could be done quickly and save time. The patient might need a clinical examination and a doctor would be assigned to do this. The list was posted in the staff room for all to see. It was a very efficient way of running a busy clinic.

But I knew we could still do more. At St Christopher's hospice in Sydenham, I had already witnessed Cicely Saunders's visionary version of patient-centred care for the terminally ill. At a time when the old authoritarian 'top-down' approach of doctors dictating treatment without involving the patient held sway, this was indeed revolutionary. I kept in touch with Saunders after I took up the oncology job in Glasgow and every six months or so went down to London to meet her and another half dozen experts in palliative care. At those meetings, for which I acted as secretary, we would discuss new techniques of both treatment and care. Just as I was inspired by such innovative ideas, so were members of my staff when I sent them down to see St Christopher's for themselves. Two of them subsequently went on to become hospice directors in their own right.

Although Ward 7B wasn't a hospice or a private charity, I had long been attracted to the notion of patient-centred care. At the leading cancer hospitals in New York and Boston I had visited in 1974 what had actually impressed me most was how the nurses seemed to have more time to chat to the patients, and make them feel more at ease.[3] But if patient-centred care meant anything, I realised, I should be doing more of it myself. I remembered the subheading of a book I hugely admired, Elisabeth Kübler-Ross's seminal 1969 work *On Death and Dying: What the Dying Have to Teach Doctors, Nurses, Clergy and their own Families*. What did the dying have to teach doctors? And when I translated that question into the work we did on Ward 7B, what did the living? What did the seriously sick think about their treatment and how could it be improved? I decided to ask a small group of cancer patients round to our house and find out.

We had moved house back in 1974 on my appointment as professor. For a while we had toyed with taking up the offer of one of the enormous four-storey houses Glasgow University had built in 1870 for its professors on a square on the main campus at Gilmorehill. One of the reasons we decided against doing so was that it didn't have a garden. Well, it did – there was a communal grass lawn at the front, although children from outside the area monopolised it. In the end, according to one story, things became so bad a sign was put up which read: 'Only Legitimate University children can play here'.

Instead, just before my youngest daughter, Susan, was born, we moved to a semi-detached house with a large garden in Anniesland Road – near enough to Knightswood for me to feel at home. It was just a short drive to the hospital, and even after I'd returned home I used to like to go back in again and check that everything was OK. I could leave my home when the first bongs sounded for the News at Ten, have a quick walk round the ward, meet key patients, speak to the staff and the nurses and be back home before the programme was over. One evening in 1978, I didn't go to visit the patients: instead, they came to visit me.

Breaking down barriers of formality can often help new ideas to develop. When William Smith founded the Boys' Brigade in Glasgow in 1884, I subsequently found out, he did something similar, inviting the boys in his troop round to his own house, where he and his wife entertained them. This, according to his biographer, was then an in-novative idea for youth and social workers like him, as while they would visit clients, 'the idea of inviting them back into their home never crossed their mind'.[4] I didn't look on inviting the meeting at our house in quite those terms, but I was keen to find out what we could be doing better, and this seemed a good way to start. Of all the things I've done in my life, starting the organisation that became Tak Tent – as we did that evening, with 20 people crammed into our lounge – is the one thing I'm most proud of. Tak Tent is the old Scots phrase for 'take care' and is used in sayings such as 'tak tent o' time ere time be tint' – take care of time or time will be lost. And I'm proud of it be-cause it was the greatest learning experience of my life.

This time, what I was learning was coming from people, not books or lectures. It was experiential. What did it feel like to be told you had cancer? Could that have been handled better? While we, in medical oncology, might be excited by the prospect of being able to turn back diseases with drugs, what did chemotherapy feel like to the patients themselves? Could their families see progress or despair as their loved one battled on? How did they explain to friends and family what was happening – and did they really understand? If not, how could we help? If they were in work – or indeed if they weren't – how were they coping? I had so many questions. I thought back to that first ever medical paper I'd written, when I had realised that some cancer patients in hospital hadn't even been told their diagnosis. Things had improved, but by how much? What did people understand about their treatment? How had other doctors told them? What information did they still need?

I wanted to find out answers because I had grown close to all the people in the room. I had seen most of them through the various stages of their cancers, from diagnosis and investigations to treatment and all the accompanying communications and conversations with the team and their families. The one thing I noticed was how keen they all were to help other patients who might still be facing everything they had already undergone. That, I realised, would be at the heart of what Tak Tent would be about – communicating how best to get through the whole experience of cancer treatment in a way devoid of 'doctorspeak', and seeing what practical steps we could each take to help each other. And we, the doctors, learnt too: no medical textbooks could possibly convey what it felt like to live with advanced cancer, for example, half as unforgettably as the character in William McIlvanney's excellent novel *Laidlaw* who says, 'It's fower-nothin' wi' two minutes to go.'[5]

It made sense to hold the first few meetings at our house, as patients, families and staff might be more inhibited in a hospital setting. Doctors, nurses, even researchers came along in their own time, and the sessions were motivating for all of us. Once everyone got to know each other, however, the setting mattered less, so we returned to the hospital. The house at the time was a busy one. Three young children, two bearded collies and lots of toys. But it was the home of a happy family. The choice of bearded collies was interesting. We had just lost our lovely flatcoat retriever Bart, and went to look at some beardies. There was a beautiful brown one and a small black one which the owner said was a runt no one would buy. We drove home thinking about what to do, and the children were furious. So we went back the following day, and bought then both, Bonnie and Clyde. In the midst of all of this I was often away leaving Ann with all five of them to look after. It was a busy time.

Everyone's reaction to cancer is different. Some people didn't want to come along to the meetings, but just wanted the information: we always respected that and just made sure we could answer all their questions. But for others, the meetings gave a sense of purpose or helped them feel less isolated – feelings which were real enough at a time when, in the world beyond the hospital, cancer was still rarely discussed and slightly taboo. Some patients became passionate fund-raisers or keen to set up their own groups. From that first meeting, Tak Tent developed to the point at which there were 30 different groups across the whole of the west of Scotland. We used the patients' experience to provide information in the form of booklets and leaflets for others, and these were often written by the patients themselves. One young woman who worked in a benefits office wrote a very useful summary about financial help; another wrote a useful piece about hair loss and where to get the best wigs. Other booklets included advice for clinic patients, guides to the various cancer treatments, or suggested diets. Back in the 1980s, cancer still had stigma attached to it, and I did my best to remove this by setting up a series of six public lectures at the university. These each attracted audiences of around 300 people and the lively discussions that followed confirmed me in any belief that the public genuinely did want to learn more. Out of this I produced a small book, *Living with Cancer*, which we sold to raise funds for Tak Tent. On it, as on all of our publications, Alexander Haddow's four-leafed Celtic knot was prominently displayed.

With the help of funding from the Cancer Research Campaign, we started Tak Tent in 1980, though it was formally launched by Lord Provost Michael Kelly at a reception in the City Chambers in November 1983. There was, as he pointed out, nothing like it in the whole of the UK. Picking up on the four needs of the whole patient that Haddow had drawn for us in his symbol – the physical, emotional, psychological and spiritual – he pointed out that the need to embrace all of them was 'fast becoming universally accepted in the medical profession' and went on to praise the social gatherings, counselling services and information services we provided such as the helpline we had introduced in Glasgow earlier that year. I was glad he mentioned that, as one of the key lessons Tak Tent had taught me was that, for all the newspaper hype about the search for a cure for cancer, too little attention was being paid to how people actually lived with the illness.

Meanwhile, we had also been breaking new ground on another

aspect of health education – and one which prefigured my work as Chief Medical Officer. It was also a project on which Ann and I could work together. Back in 1978, the Cancer Research Campaign had asked me to look at what primary school teachers were being taught about health education. I showed Ann some of the leaflets I had been given about the dangers of children smoking – a major problem in Glasgow at the time as surveys showed that as many as 15 per cent of 9–12-year-olds smoked.

She wasn't impressed. As a primary school teacher, she knew precisely how to get the message across. The leaflets, she told me in no uncertain terms, couldn't possibly do the job. 'Very well then,' I said, 'if you write something for me, I'll take it to the Cancer Research Campaign and we'll see what they think.' She did the research and wrote a proposal which was accepted. This pioneering work developed an across-the-curriculum health education programme for upper primary schools called Jimmy on the Road to Super Health which contained within it a smoking cessation programme. This was introduced to all primary schools in Glasgow as well as some in England and Northern Ireland. We also took advantage of the skills she had learnt on her postgraduate diploma in educational technology to produce video teaching materials for medical students, nurses and other professional groups.[6] In them, patients would talk about their cancer experiences – again, unremarkable now, when communication is so highly prized, but rare in the late 1970s. It was great to be working with Ann.

When I look back on my career, I realise how lucky I have been. In London, I had been privileged to meet Cicely Saunders as she pushed through a revolution in patient-centred palliative care. In Glasgow, I had been chosen, at a ridiculously young age, to be the university's first professor in a subject – medical oncology – that was just beginning, so slowly and painfully as to often hardly be apparent, to do the hitherto unimaginable, and turn back cancer. And what I was doing, as best as one man could, was to try to fuse those two different medical revolutions together.

Every year in the west of Scotland alone, there were between 11,000 and 12,000 new cases of various cancers, and yet there were only ten beds in Ward 7B. The loving-kindness, the single-minded care and attention, the lengthy conversations that Cicely and her team were able to bring to the terminally ill at St Christopher's would be impossible for us to replicate on a busy hospital ward. But that didn't mean we had to abandon the attempt. We couldn't always succeed, but we did try to treat patients with more openness and honesty than they might have found elsewhere within the hospital system. I can still remember, for example, taking a rather crowded lift to the seventh floor with a patient who asked me what his blood levels and X-rays were like. I had the latter file in my hand, so I showed him it then and there. I could see the looks of disapproval from some of my medical colleagues: there was, they clearly felt, a time and place for such discussions, and that was with the patient across the desk from the consultant. But I no longer thought like that. Tak Tent had taught me other priorities.

The sheer number of cancer patients was, however, something Tak Tent could help with. Even if I could only personally help a fraction of those 11,000–12,000 new cases, we could still try to ensure that as many as possible of the rest were also helped. The stigma attached to the disease was beginning to wane as potential treatments came in, but thousands of cancer patients no doubt still felt isolated and alone in facing up to what they wrongly persisted in seeing as a doom-laden plague. I wanted to show that they were wrong on both counts – to point out that even in the early 1980s half of all cancer cases had a good chance of doing well, that 60 per cent of leukaemias could be controlled and some other kinds of cancer (like, as we have seen, testicular cancer) had a cure rate of more than 80 per cent. Through Tak Tent's educational role, through all those booklets we had produced in the 1980s, we tried to get across the message that, at least when it came to cancer, knowledge empowered and ignorance was the very opposite of bliss.

Already, even the month before our formal launch in 1983, we were training relatives and patients to act as cancer counsellors and provide comforting advice and practical help. As the informal Tak Tent network spread, it grew to reach places as far apart as Ayrshire and Oban. Tak Tent wasn't just about self-help – the oncology department was involved at every step of the way – but it did keep patients involved in all aspects of their treatment. One of those was the extent to which they could believe the claims made on behalf of interferon as an ultra-expensive 'miracle drug' in the spring and summer of 1980. These hopes grew so wildly in the face of all evidence that Glasgow Health Board had to beg people not to phone in about it. We in the department were labelled 'medical pygmies' for wanting to see more proof of interferon's effectiveness, and some parents gave up on us and flew their children out of the city for treatment in Ireland, where they sadly died.

By 1984, I had led the department for ten years, and when another job – as ever, completely different – came up, I decided to take it. I knew I would miss many colleagues: that esprit de corps I had tried to build through the annual pantomime, the open evenings at our home, even the Golden Pisspot so often awarded for delays in getting research in on time – was real enough. Chances are, though, that I'd bump into them at some medical function or other, or find out how they were getting on through friends of friends. The patients, though: that was another matter. If they were cured, they might drive off from the Gartnavel General car park and I might never see them again, or maybe just the occasional half-remembered face at the end of a supermarket aisle or passing on the other side of the street in the rain. Where do I go to remember them?

Well, there is a place, and it is hugely important to me, so I should tell you how it came about. Tak Tent changed slightly after I left. The number of branch organisations gradually fell away, but the main ones – connected with the Western and Gartnavel General hospitals – remained strong. In 2010, we changed the charity's name to Cancer Support Scotland, and two years after that, we opened a beautifully renovated building as our main base. The cancer support centre is just a couple of hundred yards from the Beatson Oncology Department at Gartnavel, and it is so relatively modest from the outside that you might not realise how beautifully thought-out the transformation has been within. Originally built in 1904 as a chapel for the neighbouring Victorian asylum, like the best buildings, it has a kind of aura about it that fits in with its aims. It is a place of peace and calm, the complete opposite of the dark, messy confusion of cancer. Instead, it is a warmly welcoming place, where you, or your carers, can go for one of the freely available therapies downstairs (reiki, aromatherapy, Indian head massage, reflexology and so on) or talk to trained counsellors or just sit awhile and rest in the converted chapel. Somehow, a dark, leaky chapel has gained a new purpose but retained its old one of health, healing and hope. I don't know how it has happened, but it has. There is a spirituality about the building and not a sanctimoniousness. It's there in the soft green walls, the restored woodwork, Robert Anning Bell's Arts and Crafts stained glass windows above what used to be the altar (I'm biased towards the one for 'Our beloved Luke the Doctor'). Someone once said that the building 'seems to glow like a little jewel-box… the light seeming to come from within rather than without' and that's exactly how it looks to me too.

This is so obviously a place of hope and healing that it is hard to imagine that it had been closed and empty for ten years before its multi-award-winning renovation, that the roof was leaking, the interior dank and dark, and the walls bulging, the garden overgrown. It beat 900 other applicants to receive National Lottery funding, and yet that is only part of the story. The most important part is that three times more people – all in all, some 2,000 – can now be helped. So that's where I go when I want to think of the patients we helped or those whom we couldn't, and who, along with their families, gave me such great support. And as I walk up towards the building from the car park, I pass the four intertwined leaves Alexander Haddow drew up for us all those years ago. I see that emblem quite a lot when I'm inside the building – on staff T-shirts, for example, or the Cancer Support Scotland leaflets. But the one outside the main entrance to the Calman Cancer Support Centre – a place so near to where I live that I often walk the dog there – is carved in stone. It will, I'm sure, last a lot longer than me.

CHAPTER 6

Dean of Medicine

EVERY DAY THAT holiday, I took the same route. The track from the farm out to the road, then a small bit of an uphill climb from Blackwaterfoot, with Drumadoon Bay behind me. On the first day, that was pretty much all the running I did: just ten minutes, and I had all the rest of the day to spend with my family. The next day, I added on another five minutes, and the day after that five minutes more, so by the end of the three weeks, I was running for just over an hour and a half. Enough to get to Machrie and back.

On Arran, August 1983 was, right up until the end of the month, a mini-heatwave, the Azores anticyclone pushing warm air as far north as Iceland and barely moving. Even when the sun doesn't shine, there's no better country in the world than Scotland. But when it does, and when the fluttering unpredictability of our weather settles down to a rare month of sustained heat, it becomes positively paradisiacal. So on Arran that August, that meant looking out across the Kilbrannan Sound from the farmhouse we were staying in and seeing the Mull of Kintyre blurring in a heat haze beyond. It meant playing golf in my shirtsleeves with the children on the wonderful 12-hole course at Shishkine. It meant non-stop walks with the dog on Blackwaterfoot beach, skimming pebbles across the mirror-smooth sea, taking picnics in the hills. And that August, on Arran, it meant somebody who had probably never run more than two or three miles in his life training to run a marathon.

Why? It wasn't just an idle whim. My father had been 41 when he died of a heart attack, the very age I was then. I thought about him often as I ran, of how he'd missed everything about his grandchildren's lives. And maybe that's why I was running – because I wanted to live to see my children grow up and, who knew, maybe even grand-children too. Certainly, I know my father would have loved Andrew, Lynn, and Susan; and they in turn would have adored him. So as I was puffing along the road to Machrie and getting nearer and nearer with each passing day – no great distance to a regular runner, but enough of a challenge for a novice – a fairly complicated swirl of emotions rushed round my brain. Sadness for my father's too-early death and what couldn't be, but gratitude for all the good things – 'all the sweets of being', in Boswell's lovely phrase – that there already were in my own life.

One of them is Arran itself. I have loved the island ever since Ann and I first went there. Maybe it's something about that hour-long ferry from Ardrossan to Brodick just being long enough to slough off work-aday worries, maybe it's just that it's the right size of island, maybe it's the sheer variety of its 'Scotland in miniature' landscape. Or perhaps it's a case of familiarity breeding contentment and happy memories piling on each other in irresistible profusion. Whatever the reason, I felt at home there long before we bought our bungalow in Brodick. And, if I wanted any inspiration from the landscape I was jogging through, on Machrie Moor on that warm summer of 1983, it was all around me. A mile away on the moorland to the right, there was not just one neolithic stone circle but six: 5,000 years old and, even though we know little about what they were actually for, all those generations buried around about made them as good a memento mori as you could wish. Two miles in the other direction, at the bottom of sandstone cliffs above a raised beach, was the King's Cave. If you believe the legend, this was a place not of death but determination, where Robert the Bruce had his famous encounter with the spider who tried, and tried, and tried again to reach the top, finally achieving his objective. Whether or not that story is true, it's certainly inspira-tional: spiders, Scottish kings and would-be marathon runners could all draw the lesson from it that they shouldn't give up so easily.

The race itself was to take place in Glasgow on 11 September – a rare Sunday on which I skipped morning church. By the time we left Arran I was running more proficiently, but I'd still only managed about 13 miles. Now I was back at work – and there was an oncology conference in Vienna I just couldn't miss. For once in my life I was starting something with no certainty I'd be able to finish it as I wanted to. Come to think of it, though, wasn't that like life itself – especially the lives of the cancer patients I was treating on Ward 7B?

The conference in Vienna was, as if I needed any further incentive to run, all about chemotherapy. How could 'hitting the wall' possibly compare to the tougher chemotherapy regimes my patients might have to face – regimes that, with their consent, I was prescribing for them? And even if ever I did have any worries about what state I would be in as I crossed the marathon's finishing line on Glasgow Green, they dissolved completely as soon as I thought of the other question my cancer patients often asked me: 'Just how long do I have left, Professor?' My motivation couldn't be higher; no sooner was I out of the chemotherapy seminars than I was out for some last-minute training on the boulevards and in the parks of the Austrian capital.

Back in Glasgow, on an overcast, slightly blustery September Sunday in 1983, I joined 9,605 others at the mass-start of the marathon on the Saltmarket. If you had counted them all out, and counted them all back – to adapt Brian Hanrahan's phrase from the Falklands war the previous year – you would have been just six people short. Six people didn't make it all the way round the route which traced what looked like a squashed inverted ampersand over the city centre. Mercifully, I wasn't one of them. At the finishing line, we were all given a rose. It had taken me 4 hours 19 minutes and 36 seconds, which has stood as my own marathon personal best from that day to this.

Seriously, though, when I look back at my 41-year-old self running around Arran, Vienna, and Glasgow, what do I see? For a start, I remember the good health that allowed me to do so. In our Tak Tent booklet 'Living With Cancer', we did our best to define what quality of life meant. Essentially, we said, it boiled down to this: are your hopes and ambitions matched and fulfilled by experience? If my hopes and ambitions to finish the marathon weren't matched by experience – if I had been unable to finish the course due to illness, for example, or if I had been mugged at mile 17, my quality of life would have taken a knock too. In a way, that's just what had happened to my cancer patients on Ward 7B. Their expectations had taken a knock – and were now reduced – but it was our job to make sure that they were not further disappointed by the standards of care they received.

If we, as carers, could ensure that our patients were not disappointed in us, then they would have a good quality of life. If we couldn't, they wouldn't.

The quality of our cancer patients' lives mattered hugely to us: it was what we were there for. We could improve it by helping them reach the goals they'd set themselves. So we had to find out what was really important to them, and where any potential problems were. Counterintuitively perhaps, we could also improve their quality of life by reducing their expectations – which emphatically did not mean limiting hope, but making sure that their hopes were realistic. As I have already mentioned, these were exciting times for oncology. Hope was no longer in impossibly short supply. The work of people like Ken Harrap in anti-cancer drug discovery was only part of it. Combination chemotherapy was on its way in too, with the combinations being tweaked and changed so effectively that diseases like advanced Hodgkin's lymphoma – previously beyond treatment – could now be successfully reined in. There was far more than that too. Take that great British invention, the CT scanner. In 1971, the year before we moved down to Wimbledon, the world's first CT scan took place on the brain of a patient in a hospital two miles away. By 1975, EMI had introduced CT machines that scanned the whole body in 15 minutes, and the scan times were dropping all the time. By 1983, while I was trying to run a marathon in a non-embarrassing time, the CT scanner at the Western would run a whole-body scan in a minute, and unlike me, its times would get ever quicker: down to just one second in 2000. MRI (magnetic resonance imaging) wasn't too far behind: the first full-clinically useful MRI scan, at the University of Aberdeen, identified a primary tumour in a patient's chest on 28 August 1980. British scientists shared Nobel Prizes for both of these inventions – Sir Geoffrey Hounsfield for the CT scanner in 1978 and Sir Peter Mansfield, somewhat belatedly, for his work on MRI in 2003. Considering the number of lives both men's inventions have saved, it is perhaps odd that no-one seems to have yet thought to put up a statue to either of them.

Sometimes, though, when innovation is in full swing, it can be all too easy to focus on the excitement of the science rather concentrating on improving the patient's quality of life. This is where Tak Tent came in. Before it was set up, there was little in the way of mutual support for cancer patients. Organisations like Cancer Bacup or Maggie's Centres didn't yet exist. GPs could, and did, help, of course, but we should remember that the average GP, with just over 2,000 patients on his or her list, might only come across one patient with breast cancer and one with colon cancer a year, one patient with leukaemia every 15 years and one with a bone marrow tumour every 30 years. With an average of eight to ten new cancer cases a year, a GP may of course become proficient in treating such patients, but on Ward 7B this was something we were absolutely immersed in.

This didn't just mean keeping abreast of the latest scientific developments. It also involved concentrating on patients as individuals, often at a time of great uncertainty and distress in their lives. Some patients would want to know every last detail of their treatment, others might not wish to hear what was happening and deny that any problem existed. The skill of the job – its biggest challenge and biggest reward – lay in being able to communicate with each individual patient in just the right way for them. 'Bitter is truth unseasoned by grace,' St Bernard once observed. It was our job to provide that truth-seasoning grace, to show empathy and respect for their individuality and do what we could to sort out their problems and improve their quality of life.

This, of course, wasn't only my job: those aims had to be instilled in and echoed by everyone in the team. That, in turn, meant that as well as all my scientific work (for which I was elected a Fellow of the Royal Society of Edinburgh in 1979) I also took two courses at the Henley Management College. One of these was on skills appraisals, which was, in the mid-1980s, relatively new – at least in medicine – although it proved valuable in my subsequent career. What particular direction that career would take wasn't something that particularly preoccupied me. I felt fulfilled in my job and didn't have any particular ambition to do anything else. Yet when I got a phone call asking whether I would be interested in becoming Glasgow University's Dean of Postgraduate Medical Education, I was intrigued enough to apply for, and get, the job. My colleagues couldn't understand it. Why on earth did I want to leave a busy and successful clinical unit which by now had a world-class reputation and a great future? How could what was essentially an administrative job possibly be as stimulating and involving as the one I was already doing? Being postgraduate medical dean was, they implied, the kind of job I should maybe consider in my fifties or before I retired. But I was only 42, so why was I even thinking about it?

Well, as I've already said, I like a wee adventure. I love learning and finding out new things – even while in the middle of running the department of oncology in 1982, for example, I still managed to take an Open University course in Reformation Studies. I hadn't grown bored by oncology – far from it – but had always been passionate about education. When I look back on my life, it is one strand that is threaded through all of it. There were four postgraduate medical deans in Scotland, each in charge of medical training in their own region. The one I was responsible for was the west of Scotland, which, for these purposes, ranged from Oban in the north to Dumfries in the south. It contained some 1,300 higher specialist trainees, and it was my job to make sure their training was as good as it possibly could be. Innovations such as the education videos and Tak Tent itself had been well received in and beyond the department of oncology; what I wanted to do now was to encourage innovation and excellence in as wide a range of subjects as possible.

As professor of oncology, like many specialists, I had become immersed in my subject. That's inevitable: if you even took just two years away from work, you'd no longer be able to do your job properly as the knowledge base required would have expanded so far in the interim. The corollary is that for many specialists this very immersion in their own area of expertise often comes at the expense of losing touch with other areas of medicine. With my new job, I had to understand the training needed in a wide range of other subjects, from ophthalmology to orthopaedics. In that respect, it reminded me of Saturday mornings at the Western, when I was training to be a surgeon and all the junior staff – and all the consultants – would come in to hear an expert talk on latest developments in their specialism. Except, of course, now it wasn't just one hospital and a one-hour talk but improving training all the hospitals and clinics and medical establishments in the region all the time.

My friends were right about two things: it was a heavily

administrative job, and my two distinguished predecessors had both done it as their last job before retirement.[1] But for anyone with a passion for education – or who believed, as I did, that good medical education was 'the essential foundation of a comprehensive health service' – it was a wonderful opportunity.[2] It also, it must be said, provided me with one of the more imposing offices I've ever worked in and certainly the one with the best view. From my offices in the main Gilbert Scott Building at Glasgow University, I had a panoramic view over Kelvingrove Park towards the art galleries and the Clyde – and even, a couple of miles away, Gartnavel Hospital and Ward 7B silhouetted against the sunset. On the other side, I would enter from the east quadrangle, as quiet, peaceful and imposing a place as you could hope to find in the middle of a city and, in May, when the cherry trees blossomed there, as beautiful. This job, without such intense clinical work, allowed me to see the family more regularly and watch them, and the dogs grow up. The kids were progessing at school and developing wider interests, and the dogs just seemed to get dirtier than ever! I had time for the garden, and built a sandpit for the family to play in.

Although based at the university and centred on its Faculty of Medicine, the job of postgraduate dean had tremendous range. Travelling around the West of Scotland in a way that I never quite did as professor of oncology, I got to see the whole range of clinical care, from teaching hospitals with plenty of specialists to small hospitals with maybe one generalist surgeon. And as I did, I got a much clearer, wider picture of how the health of a quarter of the Scottish population was being managed – and what we still needed to do to improve it. Training courses had to be arranged for all clinical tutors, specialty advisers and chairmen of speciality sub-committees. An education committee had to be set up at all postgraduate centres, with better co-ordination with the Royal Colleges, universities and the NHS. We needed a career advisory service for all junior staff, and better computing facilities too, along with a computer database to monitor the progress of all medical postgraduates.

Then we had to take a hard look at what medical graduates really needed to learn in that hopelessly busy pre-registration year after they'd graduated with a medical degree but before full registration with the GMC. Along with Margaret Donaldson, I wrote a report-looking at what had caused hundreds of incidents involving 200 supervised junior doctors and how these could have been avoided and what lessons could be learnt from them, in terms of better teaching about priorities, greater support from senior staff, and more help with communication skills and dealing with dying patients.[3] The last of these was something particularly close to my heart as for one day a week I also worked as a consultant in palliative medicine at Victoria Infirmary. The report on junior house officers' training wasn't an entirely negative exercise, however, as we also wanted to show them the kind of issues they would be facing later in their careers and how we could make them better doctors. We also set up a series of seminars and short courses, and built up links with other education units, especially Dundee, where Professor Ronald Harden was doing great work in improving undergraduate medical education.

My predecessor, Professor Timbury, had already started work on setting up an educational research unit together with a more structured series of courses and a diploma in medical education. With proper funding, this became a department based close to the university at Lilybank Gardens which, from 1988, was able to offer MEd and MPhil degrees, as well as a Certificate in Medical Education. If such a course had been around when I was training, I'd have loved to have taken it. I would have been a much better clinical teacher if I had learnt from the best brains in the subject. Then again, I would have said the same thing about studying medical ethics. Here was another subject that not only fascinated me but which I felt had been underplayed in my own medical training. Yet issues of ethics underpinned every aspect of my clinical background, from the ethics of transplantation to judgments about quality of life in cancer treatments and palliative care. Ethics is hardly a new subject, yet in all of these issues it was suddenly looking as contemporary as robotics. No wonder, therefore, that I struck up a friendship with Robin Downie, Glasgow's Professor of Moral Philosophy, and as such the current occupant of the chair once held by Adam Smith, and subsequently collaborated with him on a number of projects. We are completely different in both our lecturing styles (he talks without either notes or PowerPoint) and intellectual background (I'd never studied philosophy in my life) yet we worked well as a kind of lecturing double-act. Together, we also started experimenting with something nobody seemed to have done before – introducing British medical students to philosophy and the arts. This has now grown into a whole new subject known as 'medical humanities'.

It all started in January 1985 when Robin and I taught a six-week course on ethics. There were about 25 students in the postgraduate medical centre and they were a particularly bright bunch. Harry Burns, about to be a surgeon at the Royal Infirmary, later to be knighted and appointed CMO Scotland, was there, and so too was Dr Jane McNaughton, soon to become a lecturer in General Practice, now Professor of Medical Humanities at Durham and one of Britain's leading lights in the subject. Among the topics we discussed were abortion, in vitro fertilisation, values in medicine, paternalism, the role of the doctor and quality of life – practical issues, in other words, not abstruse ones, and ones which we could illuminate with stories from newspapers or anonymised case histories. Or, come to that, literature.

That's what we moved onto next. It's always quite thrilling when you start teaching a course that's not quite like anything anyone has ever taught before, and that's exactly what it felt like putting together a short course on Literature and Medicine.[4] Of the two, the third-year medical undergraduates we were teaching in 1988 seemed to like the literature best, probably because of its rarity value on their curriculum. But we learnt from them as well: putting together the kind of booklists of recommended reading that would update the one Sir William Osler had produced almost a century earlier was particularly edifying. Whereas Shakespeare and Sir Thomas Browne were the only British authors on Osler's list, our students wanted to add a whole load more – *Tess of the d'Urbevilles*, *Middlemarch*, *Sunset Song* and *Cal* among them. By that stage, Robin and I had already written our first book together on medical ethics, which effectively became a textbook on the subject, Robin leading with the moral concepts involved at the start, and me bringing up a string of practical examples and ethical dilemmas in the rear.[5] I also worked alongside Professor Sheila MacLean at the university's Institute of Law and Ethics on a number of other papers on issues such as consent.[6] There was an intellectual excitement about all of this that I found quite compelling, and I still do, which is why I have been honoured to be President of the Institute of Medical Ethics and still address medical students on ethical issues. As to why the subject remains fundamentally important to me, I can turn to a moral philosopher who first taught at Glasgow University even before my own time. 'Do not expect moral philosophy to solve the practical problems of life or to be a crutch on which you can learn,' said David Raphael (1916–2015). 'A study of philosophy makes it more necessary, not less, to stand on your own feet, to be self-critical, and to be obliged to choose for yourself. It makes you more rational, more responsible, more of a human being.' I chose that quotation back in 1984 for that first evening class on ethics for postgraduate medical students. It still holds true.

One interesting aspect of my time as medical dean was an invitation to be an advisor to the Inquiry into the Dounreay nuclear plant. Sandy Bell was the Reporter and Brian Gill (later Lord Gill) and Donald MacKay (later Lord MacKay of Drumadoon) were the QCs. It began in 1986 and reported in 1987. In April that year there was an explosion in the Chernobyl nuclear power station in Ukraine and radioactivity released. While I was in Dounreay I was interested in the medical facilities available and noted that they had a whole-body radioactive counter. I thought it would be interesting to see how it felt being scanned and I did so only to find that I had some radioactive Caesium in my body from the Chernobyl incident. So far, though, I have had no health problems from that exposure.

But let's look at something else that was still only in its infancy in 1984. I have already touched on the revolution in palliative care, having witnessed its effective beginnings as a result of the work of Dame Cicely Saunders. In Scotland we owe almost as much to the work of Derek Doyle, who, in 1977, became the first medical director of St Columba's in Edinburgh, the first modern hospice north of the Border. After I became consultant in palliative care at the Victoria Infirmary in Glasgow, our paths crossed occasionally and to (I'd like to think) our mutual benefit. Previously a surgeon-missionary in South Africa, he was a man with massive experience: when he retired, he calculated that he'd worked with between 20,000 and 25,000 patients. Impossible as it might seem, such was his whole-person approach, his concern over the individual's quality of life, or how their relatives were coping, that I don't doubt that each one of them was special to him. I learnt so much from him.

In 1999, four years after he retired from St Columba's, Dr Doyle published a memoir, *The Platform Ticket*, about his life's work.[7] It gets its title from an elderly woman he met at the hospice. When he asked what he could do for her, she replied:

'Just go and get a platform ticket'. It felt strange, she explained, getting a single ticket, and while it was fine knowing that she was being looked after by a doctor with lots of fancy letters after his name, 'what I really want is a friend, and I want you to be a friend. I didn't know it was so lonely – dying is so lonely'.

Dr Doyle patted his pocket and assured her that he had his platform ticket ready to see her off. Then one day, she called him over.

She said, 'I've been waiting so long, but it's come. Have you got your platform ticket with you? Come with me.' She held my hand.

'You can't come with me all the way, but I'll feel quite safe as long as you've got your platform ticket.' She took my hand and gave it a little squeeze, and her hand dropped. And that was what, for me, it was all about. What anybody wants from their doctors at this time of life is someone who will stay by them, know their needs and their feelings and be friends to them, not just be super-highly-trained specialists.

I have quoted Dr Doyle at length because he is spot-on about the potential loneliness of death, and how palliative care can ease that final journey. The Victoria Infirmary was a 370-bed teaching hospital in the south side of Glasgow, but – just as with Ward 7B at Gartnavel – where applicable, we were keen to introduce the best practice from the hospice movement there. And just as that elderly lady had said, sometimes what we are most looking for as we approach death is just loving-kindness and simple human friendship. We didn't have a designated ward, but working as a small team alongside Dr Margaret Hutton and Sister Margaret Sneddon, we helped the staff to help the patients. It was occasionally difficult but always rewarding work.

I say 'difficult' because sometimes our patients' stories do not end as we'd hope they would, even when we try hard to do the right thing. I remember one patient, a young woman with cancer. I sat down beside her and quietly asked her whether everything was OK and put my arm on her shoulder. As soon as I had left the room, her mother came up to me. 'That was a disaster,' she said. 'She knew when you put your arm on her shoulder that her time had come.' And I felt sad that I had failed to read her thoughts correctly, because while at this stage a palliative care doctor might not be able to bring healing, there is an older medical concept of 'making wholeness'. It's not the same as curing, but it's something Derek's lady with the platform ticket felt and which – for that moment at least – my patient didn't.

In 1985, the year after I started at the Victoria, Derek helped to found the Association of Palliative Medicine, became the first editor of the new *Journal of Palliative Medicine*, and began to push for official recognition of palliative medicine as a specialism. Along with Gill Ford, the former Deputy Chief Medical Officer, who had just moved to become Director of Studies under Dame Cicely at St Christopher's Hospice, I was only too happy to help lobby the Royal College of Physicians on the new association's behalf. It worked. In 1987, Derek became the first palliative medicine consultant in Scotland, making Scotland effectively the first country in the world to create a career path for palliative medicine.

There's a coda to this story, maybe even two. Derek has always been an indefatigable writer about palliative care, and in the 2005 edition of the *Oxford Book of Palliative Medicine* – the definitive book on the subject and now used in over 100 countries – my name appears alongside his as co-editor. And more recently, on 9 July 2014, he came across from Edinburgh to Glasgow University, I waved my chancellor's cap over his head in the Bute Hall, and he instantly became a red-and-gold begowned honorary Doctor of Science. Sometimes I really love my job.

CHAPTER 7

Scotland's Doctor

ONE AFTERNOON IN the early summer of 1988, I was working in my office at Gilmorehill when the phone rang and a civil servant in the Scottish Office asked me, firstly, whether I had heard about the forthcoming vacancy for the post of Chief Medical Officer (CMO) for Scotland and, secondly, whether I would be interested in applying for it. Not only had I not heard about the vacancy, but I hadn't even heard of the job. My initial reaction was: why on earth would I ever want to be a civil servant? Why would I wish to enter a world about which I knew next to nothing? Why would I want a job without any clinical involvement whatsoever? On top of all of that, it was in Edinburgh – which, for a Glaswegian, is never exactly a plus...

But then again, my career was already full of such unpredictable moves. Why had I decided to be a surgeon when I had once seemed set on being a dermatologist? Why had I given that up for research? Why did I then take up a professorship in oncology, and why then abandon that to move into academia as postgraduate medical dean? Each of these moves was so wildly different as to make my career seem more like a game of hopscotch than any calculated, ordered progression. The one thread, through all my career moves, is that I love to learn. This, far more than money, is what motivates me. If a grossly distended bank balance was all I ever wanted, I could have taken any one of quite a number of jobs offering inflated salaries that headhunters periodically tried to tempt me with. None of them, however, would come close to matching the fulfilment I have found in repeatedly starting off in a new field, finding about the hidden challenges and complexities it contains, and sometimes even learning to think in a slightly different way as a result.

So even though I'd said I wasn't interested in applying for the job as CMO Scotland, I was mildly intrigued. What did the chief medical officer actually do? The answer, as I soon found out, was practically everything. Essentially, he or she is the nation's doctor, the one person responsible for looking after the health of the whole population.[1] There's hardly any health job with a wider remit. To work out how wide, just look at the news headlines. Each day there will be some new issue on which the CMO might be expected to either comment or to help direct government policy. To the truly effective CMO, such headlines – even when within the medical press – should not come as a surprise: the CMO is effectively at the head of a medical intelligence operation and in theory should be relied upon to have his or her finger on the pulse of new developments. In practice, this isn't always possible.

In any case, there is infinitely more about the job than responding to the day's headlines. Best practice has to be worked out and insisted upon, not only for well-established health care services but for new ones too. Government reforms – and there are so many that I used to suggest we should be issued with a medal for each one endured that we could wear at formal dinners to indicate the breadth of our experience – have to be implemented and made to work. Plans have to be drawn up to minimise infections, increase efficiencies, or improve training in fields as varied as environmental health and health education. Statistics about health care have to be analysed and comparisons made so we can identify weak points in service provision and provide remedies. From psychiatric care to dental health provision, from diabetes to diets to doctors' training, there's hardly anything that doesn't at some stage cross the CMO's desk. And then, at least every week, there's something unexpected – or, as journalists call it, news. The unexpected and the expected, the routine and the strategic, the CMO has to deal with them all. With hindsight, I am completely embarrassed that I did not know this.

It is generally accepted that there are five, often interrelated, determinants of a nation's health – social and economic factors, lifestyle, environment, the quality of its health service, and the extent of our knowledge of genetics and the basic biological mechanisms of disease – and all of them were clearly laid out in the CMO's annual report on

Scotland's health. I picked up the most recent one at the time – for 1987 – in the university library and began reading.

The report was a fascinating snapshot of both the health challenges facing Scotland and the extent to which they were being met. Its detail was consistently impressive: not only, for example, did it give the precise numbers of patients carried by ambulances (2,000,732 in 1987) but also the exact number of miles they all travelled (15,148,019). And although I had never read one before, the CMO's annual reports have, I subsequently discovered, a long and impressive lineage, beginning in 1859 when the Public Health Act required the Privy Council's Medical Officer to make an annual report to Parliament on the state of the nation's health. These – written for years by John (later Sir John) Simon, Britain's first CMO – were widely reviewed, outspoken and massively influential in ensuring that the mid-Victorian state undertook responsibility for sanitation and public health reform. The annual reports produced by the Scottish Home and Health Department were a more recent innovation. The 1987 one I found myself poring over in the university library was only the eighth.[2]

Most of the longer-term trends outlined in the report were already known to me, but they were spelled out with impressive clarity: the never-ending rise in the number of outpatients (up 11 per cent every year from 1971) and the greater numbers being treated in fewer hospital beds; the slow downward drift of neonatal deaths and deaths due to heart disease; the number of avoidable deaths due to smoking (56 per cent of deaths among men and 38 per cent among women under 44); the growing use of computers by GPs (a quarter of the practices were already using them); the rise in the number of communicable diseases due to increasing foreign travel. The report also highlighted plenty of new developments – the white paper on in vitro fertilisation, NHS building plans, approved research projects, or the introduction of new technology, such as the lithotripter to pulverise kidney stones. As I read on, I started to see the attraction of the job.

Within all of these statistics, I realised, were challenges that could be worked on. Why, for example, were more women ignoring all the health warnings against smoking? In the 1987 CMO's report, the graphs showing changes in lung cancer mortality rates couldn't be ignored. Among men, in all age groups apart from the over-75s, the overall trend was down, yet among women, in every single age category, the trend was resolutely upwards. What could be done? To what extent was this a consequence of social deprivation? What kind of message would it take to persuade Scottish women to cut out smoking?[3]

That wasn't, I hasten to say, the only reason that I decided to apply for the job as CMO for Scotland. In fact, what appealed to me was the very fact that there wasn't one single issue to deal with: this was a job with the broadest canvas of all, in which so many of the problems were interlinked, and yet there were also a whole host of ones that didn't seem to be – Lyme disease, for example, which was then appearing only in Grampian;[4] meningitis, which didn't seem to be appearing in the clusters that were being reported elsewhere, sporadic outbreaks of food poisoning, whose specific causes had to be identified and eliminated. All of these things co-existed with the bigger challenges of cancer, heart disease and AIDS, none of which had easy answers, yet for all of which I would be expected to provide Scottish Office ministers with up-to-date advice. In the first interview I gave on being appointed to the job I admitted that I didn't yet know the extent to which I would be able to influence matters, but at least there seemed to be an opportunity to do so. 'One of my functions will be to act as a facilitator – to see if things can happen outside,' I told *The Scotsman*.[5] 'One of the challenges is to try to involve other people.'

First and foremost, that meant my new civil servant colleagues at St Andrew's House, the home of the Scottish Office in Edinburgh. That first day, as I caught the train in from Scotstounhill (handily, we lived next to the station) to Queen Street in Glasgow and then on to Edinburgh's Waverley Station, I wondered how long it would take me to understand the inner workings of the civil service and how easy it would be to work together as a team with my new colleagues. My medical educational experience helped a lot: I had visited plenty of hospitals and GPs in my previous job and had some links with politicians and a few dealings with the media. My clinical experience of dealing with critical issues meant that I didn't have any worries about making decisions quickly and being able to communicate them. All of that was on the 'plus' side. Against that, though, I still had much to learn about public health and epidemiology. And the small-p political nuances of the job would, I could see even before I started the work at St Andrew's House, require a lot of care. If I was seen as being too close to ministers I would lose the trust of the medical professions; too close to the professions and I wouldn't be trusted by my minister. And what, I wondered, as the train sped towards Waverley and the coldest, longest and windiest steps out of any railway station, would it be like to work closer to the centre of power than I ever had done? To see, at first hand, how the really important decisions about health care were made? To have to know everything – everything! – about Scotland's health, and be expected to have all the facts, figures and arguments at my fingertips whenever the minister asked me?

My daughter Lynn wished to be a nurse and had enrolled in a nursing school in Glasgow. We had just arrived in Arran in the summer and found that her results in her Higher Leaving Certificate exams were better than expected, and she could get into a university to study instead. She phoned the University of Edinburgh, and there was a place available if she could get to an interview quickly. We got the ferry back straight away, off to Edinburgh for an interview and she got into the course. This meant that I could occasionally see her for a cup of tea or a pizza while I was working in Edinburgh. She was always helpful. I remember her telling me if I was going for an interview for a job then I must not do two things. First, don't say 'uningversity', that was not appropriate. And second don't go 'wooh' if the question is an interesting one. I said I would try to behave. Also, if I had to take part in press interviews I would need to be serious and answer the questions, good advice!

In the event, I made the transition to civil servant quite easily. It helped that the other medical officers in the team were consistently supportive and kept me well briefed on latest developments in their own areas of expertise – nursing, psychiatry, science, pharmacology, dentistry and the like. William (later Sir William) Reid, then head of the Scottish Home and Health Department, was a hugely important mentor to me and epitomised the very best qualities of the civil service. But there was, I realised soon enough, a collective 'mindset' whose terms I struggled to understand. The reason is simple: growing up in Knightswood, we had never played cricket. If we had done, all the metaphors civil servants used – even in Scotland – to describe their work would have instantly made sense. To me, at first, they didn't.

Later, when I started working in Whitehall, I occasionally gave speeches to my fellow civil servants in which I would gently poke fun at the extent to which they used cricketing terms – 'close of play', 'bowled a fast one', 'safe pair of hands' and so on – to describe everything they did. I would produce a standard issue civil service blue notebook from a brown envelope marked 'Confidential'. This, I would reveal, was the new civil service handbook, the so-called Cricket Book (the acronym from its title, *Centre Reviewing Information Concerning Key Elements in Terminology: Building On Organisational Knowledge*), and while I was prepared to share some of its contents, I'd have to replace it early the next day. I then went on to define some of the terms: 'played with a straight bat', for example, is 'the ability to respond to a question without answering it… an acquired skill'. Not perhaps up to my daughter Susan's stand-up standards, but I did find that this worked well, could be easily adapted to particular audiences of civil service mandarins, and even work as a management talk. What, after all, was 'winning the Ashes' but the kind of ideal outcome we were all meant to be aiming at? What was 'rolling the pitch' but sorting out problems that were likely to occur even before you held the meeting in the first place? And just in case you think that this non-cricketing Scot was pandering to his audience, when I found this book the other day, I noted that it did also contain this question: 'What's the difference between a trolley and a civil servant? Answer: A trolley has a mind of its own.' Of course civil servants had minds of their own too, even though not officially. Officially, according to guidance from the Permanent Secretary in the Department of Health, the CMO 'speaks publicly only with ministerial authority'.[6] On issues such as smoking, where I had strong views, this posed problems, but perseverance eventually won the day.

Once inside the brass doors of St Andrew's House and installed in my office overlooking Calton Hill (one thing about Edinburgh: great views) I resolved that, while I was keen to learn all I could from the team, I also needed to see at first-hand how the NHS was working across Scotland. The only way to address the conundrum of avoiding being identified with either my political masters or the medical profession, I realised, was to stay true to my values and be in constant communication with both. That meant attending lots of dinners and professional engagements up and down the country, which in turn meant that I was working exceedingly long hours and didn't see my family anything like as much as I would have liked. On the other hand, it meant that the politicians I served (Malcolm Rifkind and Iain Laing as Secretaries of State, Michael Forsyth as Minister for Health) were particularly well briefed about the NHS's needs and complexities.

But I needed briefing too, especially on public health issues, and when I started work in January 1989, there was still none bigger than the ravages caused by HIV/AIDS in housing schemes just a few miles away from my new office. This, remember, was when Edinburgh still had the reputation as 'Europe's AIDS capital' due to the high number of drug users who had contracted HIV through sharing infected needles to inject heroin – often in the so-called 'shooting galleries' in the city's peripheral housing schemes. As Edinburgh's HIV-infected drug users were overwhelmingly heterosexual, there were fears that the virus would spread rapidly into the wider community.

Less than a year before I took over as CMO, researchers had established that HIV infection rates within Edinburgh and the Lothians were running at seven times the national average, and the number of AIDS-related deaths was still rising. Of the 1,504 people in the area infected with the virus by June 1988 – a figure that had increased from 1,239 over the previous year – roughly half were drug users, a quarter had contracted it through homosexual sex and the remainder through heterosexual sex or through contaminated blood transfusion. We didn't know how many of those 1,504 people would develop AIDS, or – if they did, how long it would take, or to how many other people they would pass on the virus. Hundreds? Thousands? Tens of thousands? Either way, plans to build Scotland's first hospice for people with AIDS – Milestone House in Edinburgh, which opened in January 1991 – remained a high priority.[7] The only question was how many more of them we needed to build.

Not, of course, that we used alarmist language like that: equanimity is just as important a virtue in the public health doctor as it is among GPs. And people with AIDS already faced considerable stigmatisation, which itself could easily become an obstacle in our attempts to halt the epidemic. The challenge was to create a health education campaign that pointed out risk without engendering fear. Lothian Health Board's 1989 'Take Care' campaign, showing how HIV could be contracted and ways to prevent being infected but using the slogan 'Take care of the one you love' seemed to me to get the balance absolutely right – as well as being a neat echo of 'Tak Tent'.

By then, though, the tide in the battle against AIDS in Scotland was beginning to turn. Again, this is something that could not have been said at the time, first of all because this only emerged in hindsight, and secondly because it might seem to imply a complacency that nobody engaged in the fight ever felt. All the same, looking back, researchers found that while most HIV-positive drug users acquired the virus between 1983 and 1986, 'since then the number of new infections has declined significantly'.[8] That fact was ascribed – quite correctly in my view – to the introduction of needle exchange and methadone substitution programmes in 1986. Infection rates among HIV-positive homosexuals were found to have peaked in 1985, and although they dropped off in the mid to late 1980s remained 'relatively constant' in the 1990s. Of the three main population groups with the virus, the only increase in new infections was among heterosexual men and women – usually the non-injecting partners of drug users or travellers returning from countries with infection rates even higher than our own.

By 1989, in other words, the fight against AIDS in Scotland was a long way from being won, and its casualties – 640 Scots with AIDS by 1994 – were considerable. But the tide was being turned, and the credit for that should go to the people who were on the case even before I turned up at St Andrew's House. Dr Roy Robertson, who still runs the Muirhouse Medical Group, in one of Edinburgh's most deprived areas, played a huge role in pushing for a needle exchange programme. So too did Dr George Bath, head of Lothian's AIDS team, who died aged 44 in 1995 and who had called for such a policy to be introduced several years previously to deal with a serious outbreak of Hepatitis B. In London, Donald Acheson, the CMO England, was 'the right man in the right place at the right time'.[9] At St Andrew's House, plaudits should also go to Sir William Reid, the Secretary of the Home and Health Department, his Under-Secretary, Patricia Cox, and Dr Iain McDonald, my predecessor as CMO Scotland, who persuaded the

Lord Advocate of the necessity of the needle exchange programme. They, not me, were the ones who had faced the virus when it was at its unknowable worst. They, not me, had to contend with its deadly ravages before the first test for it became available in 1985. They, not me, had persuaded a Conservative government to deal with injecting drug-users in a way that was at variance with its natural inclinations.

I didn't realise it, that summer's day in the university library, when I read the CMO Scotland's annual report for 1987, but all too soon I would be at the centre of the government's fight against an epidemic that was every bit as deadly.

Bovine spongiform encephalopathy (BSE) only became a notifiable disease in June 1988. When I became CMO Scotland and wrote up, in the following year's annual report, the infections that needed to be kept under surveillance, there was still no evidence as to whether it posed any health risk to humans. As the disease's incubation period was thought to be between four and five years, I estimated that 'it would be 1992 at the earliest before we knew this'. All the same, its similarity with Creutzfeldt-Jacob disease in humans was obvious from the start and research had shown that it could be transmitted to mice. We were right, it turned out, to be worried.

In July 1988, a month before the announcement that I was to be Scotland's next CMO, the government ordered the destruction of the whole carcass of any animal infected with what was already becoming known as 'mad cow disease'. On 1 January 1989, milk from infected cows was ordered to be destroyed and the protein content of cattle food reduced. Officially, that was also the day I started working as CMO. One way or another, mad cows were going to follow me around for a long while yet.

CHAPTER 8

London Calling

I'D NEVER HEARD of Saxton Bampfylde, but I guessed that they were a pharmaceutical company, so when they rang one afternoon in 1991 I told my secretary I couldn't speak to them. They phoned back, and got the same message. Only on their third call did they mention that they were actually a multinational firm of head-hunters, and a well-known one, and were currently putting together a list of candidates for the job of Chief Medical Officer for England. Would I be interested in applying?

I wasn't sure. I was only in my third year as CMO Scotland, and many of the projects I had set in motion were still unfinished. To take just one example, there were still 600 medical audits underway into the effectiveness of Scotland's doctors, and I was looking forward to finding out, and implementing, their conclusions. True enough, Ann and I had been talking about making a change, but that only involved looking at whether or not we should buy a flat in Edinburgh. We had never thought about leaving Scotland, because why would we? We had both been born, reared and educated here. We both love Scotland, nearly all our friends were here, and so were nearly all the projects we had worked on. Why move?

There were two other reasons for caution. Being an effective CMO – essentially, not only trying to nudge a whole country towards better health but also making sure the entire medical profession is doing its best to help it do so – is a hugely demanding job. A key part of it involves trying to persuade millions of people to overcome their inherent akrasia, which means knowing what they are doing is wrong, but continuing to do it.[1] Smoking is a classic example: by now most smokers surely know that their habit is not good for their health, yet they still refuse to quit. The challenge – and it is one that is close to my heart for obvious reasons – is to devise a strategy that will override smokers' akrasia.

Because public health involves so many other departments – environment, education and housing, to name just some of the more obvious – without widespread co-operation, meaningful change is impossible to effect. And without the active support of one's colleagues in the medical profession, it is pointless to even try. So while I was flattered to be asked to take the job as CMO England, I could see straight off that there was a strong argument that I would be a lot more effective as CMO in Edinburgh than I would ever be in London. At St Andrew's House in Edinburgh, the top civil servants from different departments were all in the same building, and as they already met informally, bringing about wide-ranging policy shifts was a lot easier than it would be among the bigger, separate, and often rival departmental bastions of Whitehall. And while I would hope to have the active support of my colleagues if I took the job in England, this might take time to build up. In Scotland, by contrast, I already knew all the key players, having deliberately set aside two days a week to travel around Scotland to find out their needs and explain more about our own ones. On top of that, of course, as postgraduate dean I had already supervised 350 medical teaching jobs and been responsible for the training of 6,000 more medics. In short, they knew me in Scotland; in England, while I wouldn't exactly be starting from scratch, it would be a lot harder.

So, when I talked things over with Ann that night, we tried to weigh up those two different futures. In one, maybe we would buy a flat in Edinburgh's New Town and I could jog round Arthur's Seat before turning up for work at St Andrew's House. I'd be closer to my family who were still all living in Scotland. I would work doing a job I enjoyed in a country I loved until I retired. Yes, maybe I would always wonder whether I should have applied to be CMO England, and yes, I still liked a wee adventure, but of all the job changes I had ever considered or made, this would actually be the least radical. So why even bother?

And then there was the other future. London. And because it was so much more unknowable and unpredictable, in the end, I went.

My last day at St Andrew's House was Friday 13 September 1991, and the headlines in that day's newspapers told me exactly what issue would be dominating my in-tray when I started work as CMO England on Monday morning. In his final press conference, which was meant to be about his annual report, Sir Donald Acheson had mentioned that a monthly breast self-examination 'does not reduce the risk of a woman dying from breast cancer' and may even give a false sense of security. The newspapers picked up on this because it contradicted the advice that the Department of Health had been giving for years, and this immediately led to a flood of complaints from breast cancer surgeons, cancer survivors, women's groups and many more. Anger was widespread and understandable.

Sir Donald's arguments about the inefficacy of breast self-examination did, however, have statistical support. Two years previously, an extensive longitudinal study on the efficacy of self-examination in the early detection of breast cancer involving 63,000 women, had found no real difference between women who were offered training in breast self-examination, and given a referral clinic, and a control group.[2] It seemed counter-intuitive, but subsequent large-scale studies yielded the same results. Obviously, we couldn't argue against evidence-based science, but nor did we want to dissuade women from taking responsibility for their health.

Over my years in Whitehall there were countless occasions like that, when the CMO's guidance was sought on controversial or newsworthy matters. This was part of the job: each day Parliament was sitting, for example, my department had to deal with a huge number of parliamentary questions – in 1993, the daily average was 28 – and many of these involved contentious subjects. Although I didn't deal with all of these personally, I bore ultimate responsibility for ensuring that we provided correct guidance on health matters raised in the 25,560 letters we received from MPs and 58,600 from members of the public that year.[3] Readers will doubtless be relieved to find out that I don't propose to plod through every single topic from those postbags that did manage to reach my desk, but breast self-examination – or BSE as we called it back then before bovine spongiform encephalopathy got hold of the acronym – was the first one I had to deal with when I arrived in my new job, so perhaps I should explain in a little bit more detail how I tried to handle the controversy. After all, as *The Guardian* pointed out at the time, it was indeed a 'vivid demonstration of the dangers CMOs face in their tightrope walk determining health management'.[4]

First, some background. Sir Donald Acheson had served his country well in his time as CMO, and I was hugely disappointed on his behalf that the controversy overshadowed the overall picture of the country's health unveiled in his farewell report, which was, to a large extent, a record of achievement. It also occluded proper appreciation of his successes in his eight years as CMO, not least the way in which he doggedly pushed radical public health policies that kept the AIDS epidemic at bay. On a personal level, he had been very helpful: for the three days before that fateful press conference, we had both been attending the World Health Organisation European region meeting in Lisbon, where he not only introduced me to the main delegates but assiduously explained the importance of the international dimensions of the CMO's job.

In my first week, though, it was the domestic dimension that dominated, and on my fourth day in the job I summoned experts on breast self-examination to a meeting in Oxford. The problem, we soon realised, lay in the inadequacy of the data. Only a small minority of women routinely examined their breasts for tumours, nor was there any consensus over what constituted competent self-examination or how often this should be carried out. Variations in techniques of self-examination were widespread and confusing and, as one of our experts pointed out, evidence showed that the more numerous, complex and unpleasant the procedures involved, the less likely women were to remember to do them. Many women didn't even want to learn the techniques involved, whether because of anxiety over finding any lumps or fear of unnecessary worry and the risk of needless operations. Even in the early detection survey mentioned earlier, trial acceptance rates at the two centres offering breast self-examination training were only 35 per cent and 53 per cent.

The irony is that when it came to breast screening – as opposed to breast self- examination – Britain really did have a lot to celebrate. In 1987 we had become the first large country in the world to offer a comprehensive breast cancer screening programme. Every woman aged between 50 and 64 was offered a three-yearly mammogram, as part of a programme offering a full diagnostic service and in-built evaluation studies. Ten per cent of these produced results suggesting the need for further evaluation, and only five per cent of those re-examinations would identify cancers, so many women inevitably had to suffer what might well turn out to be needless worry. But the potential gains were enormous. As Sir Donald himself had pointed out in a lecture three years previously, all the evidence was that the new programme would save thousands of lives.[5] In this, he drew a comparison with the cervical cancer programme introduced in 1966, which 'in spite of the completion of tens of millions of smears and the expenditure of tens of millions of pounds' had produced 'precious little to show for it. There has been only a small reduction in the mortality from cervical cancer and in spite of our efforts over 22 years about half of the cases of cervical cancer presenting for treatment are in women who have never been screened.'

At our Oxford meeting it soon became clear that breast self-examination was not going to match the 30 per cent reduction in mortality that the breast screening programme then looked likely to deliver and would more likely mirror the much poorer record of the cervical smear programme. In the conclusions of one of the papers we considered, 'the specificity of BSE as a screening test is low, and the cost in terms of false positive results, anxiety, suffering and the use of medical resources may be high'.[6] Five days later, we held another meeting of experts, this time at Richmond House, the Department of Health's base overlooking the Cenotaph in Whitehall. Round the table were some of the world's leading experts in breast cancer – people like Professor Roger Blamey, who had turned Nottingham into a major centre for breast cancer screening and research; Professor Sir Patrick Forrest, a fellow Scot and a former Chief Scientist in Scotland whose report led to the establishment of the NHS's breast cancer screening programme; Professor Paddy Boulter, whose research in Guildford paralleled Forrest's in Edinburgh; and Professor Michael Baum, a pioneering breast cancer surgeon then at King's College London. Again, the consensus was clear, and the next stage was to meet the minister and take the matter further, which I did the following day.

I had already been introduced to the minister, Virginia Bottomley, on my second day at Richmond House. Civil servants aren't supposed to have favourites, but in my time in Whitehall she was probably the one who impressed me the most. The fact that she was actually a Scot (born in Dunoon) had nothing to do with it. As well as that inbuilt natural advantage, though, she also had an ability to pick up complex issues remarkably quickly, and in our meeting about breast self-examination that was immediately obvious. The scientific evidence didn't warrant supporting monthly self-examination, but the political imperative was to avoid any appearance of a policy U-turn, and the public health reality was to avoid discouraging women (or men, come to that) from taking an active interest in their own health. All of this, as you can appreciate, was a fairly complicated balance of priorities, yet one which Mrs Bottomley grasped straight away. So when I phoned up Sir Donald the next day – Friday 27 September, the end of my second week in the job – to let him know how things were progressing on the breast self-examination front, I was confident enough to reassure him that things were going well.

Let's pause there for a second. Already, perhaps, you can see from this one example, some of the inherent difficulties of the CMO's job. First of all, and above everything else, comes responsibility to the public: from Sir John Simon's 1855 appointment as Medical Officer to the General Board of Health onwards, protecting the public's health – in his case, primarily through sanitary reform – has been the whole point of the job. With breast cancer, that meant doing our utmost to fight a potentially fatal disease, then being diagnosed in almost 25,000 British women a year and causing the deaths of 15,000 of them; it meant not discouraging them from looking after their own health but not wasting their time on ineffective methods of prevention either. Secondly, there's a responsibility to science, and by extension, the medical profession. Nothing Sir Donald had said was not backed by evidence-based research. Thirdly, there was a responsibility to the politicians I served but – yet another tightrope here – to whom I had to offer absolutely independent advice. Finally, as head of all the medical staff in the Civil Service (the post ranks as the equivalent of a Permanent Secretary), the CMO has a managerial responsibility to the staff he or she leads. In those two weeks, when I was beginning to get to know my colleagues, it was this aspect of the job that took up by far the most of my time. Adviser, administrator, publicist, co-ordinator, doctor: even in my first two weeks I could see the job had many roles and a cat's cradle of masters. I was working ridiculously long hours, but I loved it.

Or at least I did until I opened The Sunday Times that weekend. I'd been told what to expect after my pager went off on Saturday night, but it was still dispiriting to see the story in black and white. The government was about to make a complete U-turn on breast self-examination, the newspaper said, in a story accompanied by a cartoon of Sir Donald that was both unfair and vicious. He phoned me to ask whether the experts we'd spoken to that week had raised any queries about what he had said. No, I told him; we were as dismayed as he was by the coverage and hoped it would be forgotten as soon as possible, which is why we refrained from making any further statement. In any case, Mrs Bottomley would be fronting a press conference on the whole matter in two days' time at which our new policy would be announced.

Instead of urging women to check their breasts at a specific time each month according to a set technique, the new policy of 'breast awareness' launched at the press conference encouraged them to check their breasts on convenient occasions such as when dressing or bathing. If done regularly enough and at different times of the month, obvious changes could be noted and reported. It was a classic compromise: we weren't rebutting what the research was telling us about the unreliability of self-examination in terms of cancer prevention, but we also wanted to send a signal of encouragement to all those women who paid close attention to their own health. Breast self-examination had, after all, been recommended policy for the previous 60 years; for women in the 50-plus age group most at risk, it was advice they might have heard from their mothers and maybe even their grandmothers, perhaps one of the few pieces of health advice that had leapt across from generation to generation of women without apparently being contradicted by science. It wasn't only because of this that many women passionately believed in it, and there were indeed plenty of breast cancer survivors who vociferously insisted that they owed their lives to the practice. Drill down into current research projects and there were even hints that women taught self-examination techniques had slightly smaller tumours and less axillary spread (ie to their armpits) than those who hadn't been taught.[7] Dismissing the value of self-examination altogether seemed, in terms of public health, counter-intuitive – at least for now.

The guidelines were also changing on an even more emotive topic. Within two months of starting the job, I had summoned a group of experts to consider new evidence about how best to reduce cot deaths. In the previous decade, evidence had been mounting that putting infants to sleep on their fronts, parental smoking, and infant overheating were all likely risk factors. Evidence from New Zealand was particularly strong.[8] Alarmed at its high cot death mortality rates, health authorities there had commissioned a three-year case control study – then the biggest of its kind – into the disease. This ended in 1990 and its conclusions were clear from the start: 72.7 per cent of cot death victims slept on their stomachs and 66 per cent had mothers who smoked. In March 1991, the New Zealand government launched a major public health prime-time TV campaign in which parents were urged to place sleeping babies on their backs. This accelerated an already sharp decrease in mortality rates.

In July 1991, the four-month-old son of British television journalist Anne Diamond was found dead in his cot. Distraught, she set out to find out more about cot death and soon came across the evidence from New Zealand suggesting that sleep position was a likely factor. This also accorded with the conclusions of a small-scale project in Bristol, which had ended that month and which also suggested a causal connection between the two.[9] When Ms Diamond, who had by then returned from New Zealand, where she had interviewed key figures in their cot death prevention programme, asked what steps the Department of Health was taking, I took the advice of our own leading experts. There was indeed, they concluded, 'no evidence that placing healthy babies on their back resulted in an increased risk from choking or vomiting'. This was, of course, the main fear, and because (again, like breast self-examination) it seemed to intuitively make sense, it had become accepted practice in the 1950s, when it received the imprimatur of US parenting expert Dr Benjamin Spock. Our recommendation that babies be placed on their backs to go to sleep was made in a press release and letter sent out to all doctors, nurses, mid-wives, and health visitors on 21 November 1991 and our advice in relevant health education booklets was changed accordingly. As long as the underlying causes of cot death remained unexplained, we said, it would remain with us, but the risks of it happening could be reduced. The importance of babies sleeping on their backs remained paramount, but we stressed that this wasn't the only risk factor: cigarette smoke and infant overheating were also important. That last point was actually mentioned in the *This Week* documentary Ms Diamond made, but seemed to somehow get lost in subsequent media coverage.

After Ms Diamond's documentary was screened, its message further amplified by the many moving interviews she subsequently gave about a cause so clearly close to her heart, and the December 1991 launch of the department's 2 million pound 'Back To Sleep' campaign, Britain's cot death figures started to tumble too. In March 1991, there were 321 in England and Wales. A year later, this number had dropped to 128. According to cot death charity The Lullaby Trust's latest figures, the incidence of Sudden Infant Death Syndrome has dropped by 78 per cent since 'Back to Sleep' began. I wanted to see that figure drop even more, so when investigative reporter Roger Cook made a documentary (*The Cook Report*, broadcast on 14 November 1994 by Carlton TV) linking cot deaths and the effect of mould on fire-retardant chemicals used in baby mattresses, I commissioned another expert group. Four years later, their final report echoed their interim one in 1995 that there wasn't any evidence to back up the theory.

The 'Back to Sleep' campaign was officially launched just three months after I first started work at Richmond House as CMO England. In that time, I was so busy I was hardly ever at the house we'd bought at Sydenham, and often whole months would pass before I got the chance to eat there. Ann had remained back in our Glasgow house and I would get up there for a weekend whenever I could, or she would come down to London. But if I was alone at the Sydenham house, every Sunday night I would prepare for the next week's work. On the sofa, I'd lay out the papers and slides I needed for the next day's meetings and the suit, shirt, tie and shoes I'd wear each day for the rest of the week. I am a bit obsessive! First thing in the morning

– always early because I insisted on being at my office by 7.30am – there it all would be, waiting for me. Outside, my driver Tony would be waiting too – a really pleasant, helpful man whose company I always enjoyed – and off we'd go to, well, who knew what? I've already mentioned two of the more obvious changes I made in health policy, but the ones I really wanted to make were deeper, more structural. They were about communicating better and providing leadership – the kind of things that don't make headlines but which people can respond to and feel motivated by. I wasn't arrogant enough to think that I had all the answers, but I think at least I had some of the questions right. And for that, I think I owe a lot to those ethics classes I taught with Professor Robin Downie back in Glasgow, where we tried to help medical students analyse the kind of problems they might encounter in their everyday work.

As I was writing this, I chaired a seminar/discussion group of around 70 medical students, on the subject of ethics in medicine and science. I presented them with a series of topics/questions for them to discuss in small groups and then to report back to the wider group. This would illustrate if there were any differences in views. These related to issues which might be raised with the CMO or with health-related organisations, including those related to the medical profession such as the BMA, the Medical Royal Colleges, the General Medical Council, and with ministers. The questions included:

Should people over the age of 70 should be tagged in case they get lost?
The cost of treating and small group of patients with rare disease is often very expensive. Is this a good use of public money?
Should cigarette smokers be denied treatment on the NHS?
If you found a source of 2 million pounds to use on the NHS and you could spend it on children or the elderly, which would you choose?
If you were an MP/MSP and there was to be a debate on assisted suicide, what information would you need to help you decide on your own position?

The students discussed these questions with real vigour and showed how they could come to decisions based on evidence and on values. These discussions with the students on such issues often clarified my own thinking.

I'm going to say nothing at all about my own answers to those questions, nor did I tell the students what to think.[10] But a whole host of questions I found myself thinking about while Tony drove me to work in Whitehall were just like that. Not the same, obviously, but they were similar in that they were about real-life problems and real-time resources. Clarity in the smaller picture gives you clarity in the bigger one too. Those ethics classes buttressed my decision-making more than I realised at the time. I can't remember whether I have ever properly thanked Robin Downie for what I learnt from him, but in case I haven't, I do now. And meantime, three other students whose views were absorbing were my children, who all graduated from university during this time, and I was so proud of them. I even managed to attend all the graduation ceremonies! They mean so much to me, and their careers have made me realise just how much talking with them and discussing what they are doing, gives me such pride and pleasure.

CHAPTER 9

Mad Cows

ON THE WALL of the meeting room of my office in Whitehall, there was a print of what either is, or ought to be, the most famous cow in the world. She was called Blossom, lived on a farm near the Gloucestershire village of Berkeley, and in May 1796, she had contracted cowpox, a viral disease of the udder. When milked by hand, this can be contracted by humans, and that's exactly what had happened to the woman who milked Blossom and who then went to ask the local doctor whether there was anything he could do to help. She was right to be worried: cowpox was a less virulent strain of smallpox, but the symptoms looked similar. And in the English countryside at the end of the 18th century, there was a one in ten chance that smallpox would kill you. The local doctor she consulted was Edward Jenner, whose pioneering work on vaccination is often said to have saved more lives than that of any other human being. On 22 April 1996, I visited his splendid Georgian house – now turned into a museum – and saw the thatched rustic hut at the bottom of his garden in which Jenner treated the poorer families of the district. He called it the 'Temple of Vaccinia', and it was here that he conducted the experiments in cowpox vaccination – a neologism he coined himself from the Latin word vaccinus, meaning 'from the cow' – which he could prove offered protection against smallpox.

Jenner's thatched hut has been called 'the birthplace of public health', and 200 years after his experiments with Blossom's cowpox, it seemed a particularly apt place to visit. The BSE crisis – bovine spongiform encephalopathy, another cow-related disease – was at its height. As CMO, I was in the eye of the storm. It dominated my life.

As the years pass, some people might forget the devastation the

BSE crisis wrought on British agriculture, or the terrible cost in human lives of variant Creutzfeldt-Jacob Disease (VCJD). I never will. The causes of both diseases have been examined by the Phillips Inquiry at the kind of length (3,000 files, 300 witnesses, a 16-volume final report) I do not propose to replicate, and the science underpinning the whole topic is explored in admirable depth in several books as well as a freely available OpenLearn course run by the Open University.[1] Here, however, I shall confine myself to a narrower, but still important topic: how does the CMO handle a public health disaster of such magnitude? And what lessons can be learnt from it that will help us cope when another one comes along – as it surely will?

First of all, some (very brief) background. In March 1996, we realised that we were dealing with the entirely new disease of VCJD in which humans developed a fatal degenerative brain condition as a result of eating meat from cattle with BSE. The crisis has been building up since at least 1986 when a pathologist at the Government's Central Veterinary Laboratory examined the brain of a cow from a Sussex farm which died of a disease the local vet had never seen before. We have known about spongiform encephalopathy (in which the brain examined on autopsy, appears to have developed tiny holes, causing it to appear like a sponge) in humans since Creutzfeld-Jacob Disease was first described in 1920. In sheep, a similar disease has been known about since 1732 – called 'scrapie' because one of the clinical signs of the condition was that the affected animals compulsively scraped off their fleece against walls, rocks and trees. In all those years though, there has never been any suggestion that scrapie was transmissible to humans, and so when what looked like its bovine equivalent made its first appearance, many people thought that this would be the case with BSE too.

In the late 1980s, the numbers of cattle dying from this new disease kept rising: a mere six positive cases and 13 suspected ones in May 1987 had shot up to 600 probable cases by May 1988. In March 1988, Sir Donald Acheson, my predecessor as CMO England, was asked by the Ministry of Agriculture, Fisheries and Food (MAFF), to rule on whether BSE posed any risk to humans. He acted quickly. Within 25 days he had summoned all the relevant experts to meetings at which they decided what course of action the scientific evidence indicated should be taken. All options were on the table, from no action at all to a complete ban on beef, but the unanimous view was that an advisory group needed to be formed to keep the topic under review. Sir Donald also took advantage of the nine o'clock Wednesday morning meetings chaired by Cabinet Secretary Sir Robin (later Lord) Butler of all the departmental permanent secretaries to brief them about this potential threat to the nation's health.[2] Those weekly meetings are at the very core of this country's government, often providing the highest echelon of the civil service with their first glimpse of the problems or opportunities they might face in coming months. Later I would use them myself to alert my colleagues to similar potential risks.

The independent expert advisory group was set up under the chairmanship of eminent scientist Sir Richard Southwood, whose report in February 1989 allowed Acheson to conclude that 'the risk to Man has been extremely small and that... every reasonable step has already been taken to minimise any theoretical risk of transmission by destruction of affected cattle'. The report did, however, recommend that further research into BSE should be carried out by a group of experts led by the distinguished virologist David Tyrell. This in turn led to the formation of a standing committee, the Spongiform Encephalopathy Advisory Committee (SEAC), which met regularly throughout the BSE crisis, and which provided me with the scientific advice I needed. It also led to the creation of the National CJD Surveillance Unit, based at the Western General Hospital in Edinburgh, which had the specific job of checking whether there was any change in the pattern of CJD that might be attributable to human infection with whatever was causing BSE in cattle.

By 1990, then, even though much about BSE remained unknown and the number of cases was still rising, we thought our defences against it being transmitted to humans were in place. As early as 1987, the probable cause of the disease had been identified as infectious proteins, called prions, in meat and bone meal fed to cattle. This feed had been banned, and now, as a further consumer protection measure, not only were all animals showing symptoms of BSE slaughtered, but (in November 1989) all high-risk bovine offal – brain, spinal cord and spleen – was taken out of the human food chain. All milk from cows in which the disease was suspected had already been ordered to be destroyed the previous year.

As CMO Scotland, my annual reports reflected this increasing concern. The one for the year ending December 1989 mentioned BSE, but only in passing, noting that the incidence of the infection in Scottish dairy herds was lower than in England.[3] Compared to coronary heart disease, smoking, HIV and implementing NHS reforms, it was a low priority. By 1990, though, it was beginning to be more important. Even if it was a purely epizootic disease (one affecting only animals), it was becoming a significant one. The numbers of infected cattle throughout Britain seemed to be rising exponentially: 21,922 by the year's end, including 694 in Scotland.[4] In May that year there had been a further alarm when a dead cat in Bristol was found by a scientist at the Central Veterinary Laboratory to have died from a disease that was remarkably similar to BSE, or quite possibly BSE itself. I was at a WHO meeting in Geneva with Sir Donald at the time when he was given the news. The disease was also found in zoos in a number of wild animals fed with meat and bone meal, and the infection was introduced experimentally into a number of other species, including pigs. If the concern with BSE was that, as 'bovine scrapie', it had already jumped across one species gap, here was evidence that it could leap across some more.[5]

Hindsight, of course, is always 20:20, but in fairness to my colleagues at the Ministry of Agriculture, Fisheries and Food (MAFF), within a year of identifying an entirely new disease and working out its likely transmission route, they had set up a system that theoretically should have closed it off. The Tyrell Committee, tasked with investigating whether the transmission of BSE to all of those other species in experiments posed any threat to human health, decided that it did not and that there was no risk from eating beef. A House of Commons Select Committee came to the same conclusion. For a while, we in Scotland worried about BSE and dogs. Before MAFF set up the specified bovine offal ban (brain, spleen, spinal cord, thymus, tonsil and intestine) might dogs have been eating such infected meat? Just in case, we in Scotland ordered a survey. The Medical Research Council also set up a committee of experts to co-ordinate research into transmissible dementias in humans. But what we really needed to find out whether the disease was transmissible to humans were three things:

proof that there was a new disease, or a change in its incidence, or a test for it in humans. And in 1990, all of this was a long way off, yet my annual report for the year as CMO Scotland sounded a note of ultra-cautious optimism. Indications were

> that present levels of cases would continue in 1991 with, hopefully, the beginning of a decline in 1993. There was no conclusive evidence of vertical or horizontal transmission.

That's exactly how the graph of confirmed BSE cases looked too. A sharp rise in 1992, then a substantial fall in the next successive years.[6] The graph for cases of variant CJD – the new human disease which we didn't yet know about – didn't look like that at all. Or rather, it did, but with a five-year delay. For the first five years, it waited invisibly in the shadows, beyond the reach of our science.

I moved down to London to take up the CMO's job in September 1991 and, as mentioned in the last chapter, was soon immersed in issues such as breast cancer self-examination and cot deaths. Just to give some indication of the range of health issues I found myself looking after, I should point out that in the last three years of his tenure, Sir Donald Acheson had set up no fewer than 31 committees (SEAC was just one of them) and he also regularly attended a series of nine other meetings, for example the Wednesday morning one with the permanent secretaries. I was every bit as busy but, in course of my tenure, the number of medical staff in the department halved due to 'rationalisation'. That said, the ones I did have were superbly efficient and committed and I couldn't have asked for better.

Towards the end of my first year in the job, in August 1992, I was told about a farmer who was suspected of having CJD. When he died in February 1993 and the autopsy confirmed that he had indeed died of the disease, I consulted the Spongiform Encephalopathy Advisory Committee who assured me that there was still no scientifically proven link with BSE and that it was therefore still safe to eat beef. The following year, I received the same advice in connection with the illness and then death, apparently from CJD, of a 16-year-old girl. The press had been speculating that infected meat in hamburgers was to blame. Again, I repeated the experts' advice.

If I'd known then what I found out in October 1995, I'd have been a lot less certain about that advice – indeed, I wouldn't have given it at all. I had always assumed that arrangements MAFF had set up in abattoirs to separate potentially infective material from meat for human consumption were working as promised. On 23 October 1995 a letter I received from the Chief Veterinary Officer told me that this wasn't the case: spot checks on abattoirs had found four carcasses in which the spinal cord had not been properly removed. This was, I was told, 'unfortunate'. I thought it was a lot worse than that.

I have always believed in utter transparency in matters like this; only by pointing out potential health risks where they are known and proven to exist can we avoid the appearance of subterfuge and cover-up even when (as here) it doesn't exist. In a memo to ministers to explain what had been found at the abattoirs, I was keen to flag up the potential risk to human health this revealed. To the MAFF officials this was 'a step too far'; instead they wanted to highlight that there was still not a single case in which specified bovine offal had entered the human food chain. In the end, the agreed text did mention that what had been uncovered in the unannounced abattoir inspection was a potential health risk but added that there was still no evidence that the human food chain had actually been compromised.

The division of responsibilities between the departments had been clear from the start, with anything pertaining to animals (abattoir standards and inspections, for example) the responsibility of MAFF, and matters to do with human health falling under the jurisdiction of our own department. Personally, I always got on well with my opposite number in MAFF, but we made sure that there never was any doubt over the primacy of human health over farming interests. On a couple of occasions during the BSE crisis my CMO colleagues and I agreed that we would collectively resign if a particular policy line was taken. In neither case did we even threaten to do so, or go as far as informing ministers of our concern, as the decisions they made went in our favour.

After further investigations uncovered yet more failings in the abattoir and feedmill checkups, on 7 November, I told Douglas Hogg, the Minister for Agriculture, that I was no longer prepared to provide the kind of assurances about the safety of British beef that I had done in the previous two years. I also helped to push through the ban on mechanically recovered meat – the scraps blasted off abattoir carcasses by high-pressure hoses – which came into effect in December 1995.

And so to 20 March 1996, when BSE changed from crisis to cataclysm. Before then, 160,000 cattle with the disease had been slaughtered, along with 30,000 in which it was suspected. Afterwards, that number soared to 3.3 million. Before March, there had been no clear scientific support for the notion that BSE was transmissible to humans. Now there was, and there were alarming estimates about the new disease of variant CJD's likely death toll: up to 130,000, according to one mercifully over-pessimistic prediction. (The actual number of deaths due to variant CJD since 1995 is 178 [in 2019]; although there haven't been any for the last three years, it would be wrong to be complacent, as a further spike in the figures cannot be ruled out.)[7]

Looking back on my diary for the month, it is interesting to see how events lead up to and flow from that pivotal moment at 3.31pm on 20 March when Health Secretary Stephen Dorrell got up from the front bench in the House of Commons to announce that a new variant of CJD had been identified in young people and this was now thought to have probably been caused by eating BSE-infected meat before the introduction of the offal ban in 1989. At the start of the month, there were the usual plethora of meetings that are the lot of the CMO: a hospital in Bath had to be visited and a speech given; a circular on confidentiality to be prepared; talks held with European CMOs and a WHO regional director; staff welfare issues to be discussed; a new agenda to be set for A&E; and (just for once, not on official business) a retiral dinner for a colleague to attend in Glasgow.

The first hint that we would have to change our policy on BSE came on Monday 11 March, when I was told that SEAC thought that a cluster of cases of CJD occurring in people aged under 40 had a distinct pathological pattern. It looked as though our worst fears were becoming true. Over the next few days, as we waited for greater clarity from SEAC, we began to formulate our policy response in a series of meetings involving both Agriculture Minister Douglas Hogg and Mr Dorrell. By the following Monday, 18 March, these meetings were starting to take over my diary. Yet when I look back, what strikes me is just how many other topics had to be dealt with too. That day was a case in point. I had two meetings with Mr Hogg and Mr Dorrell – in the morning, to prepare a letter about the crisis for them to send jointly to Prime Minister Major and in the evening a lengthy session on the detailed policy response. On top of that there was huge meeting on CJD with NHS experts, vaccine specialists, medical regulatory agencies and the department's press officers, and a separate meeting with the CMOs for Scotland, Wales and Northern Ireland. Somehow, all the other business of the day had to be fitted in too, which meant that I also attended a briefing and press conference on cervical cancer screening, liaised on smallpox policy with a leading American physician; held a difficult meeting about problems in the cardiac surgery unit of the Bristol Royal infirmary; and another one on the Medical Research Council's stocktake.

That night I went home to bed, got up at 6am and by 6.30am had a draft statement ready. The story had leaked overnight – OFFICIAL: MAD COW CAN KILL YOU announced the banner headline on the front page of the *Daily Mirror* – but at least we now had a coherent policy in place, which the two Ministers would announce that afternoon. By 8.00am SEAC had agreed to the wording, and I set off for No. 10 to present it to the Cabinet and answer questions. Considering the sheer awfulness of the news we had to impart, from a purely presentational point of view, the rest of the day went well enough, with a huge, well-handled press conference in the Queen Elizabeth II Centre in Westminster. In the House of Commons, Dennis Skinner, picking up on my remarks that I would continue to eat beef as part of a balanced diet, joked that I was laying down my life for my country. A number of journalists phoned my daughter Lynn, a vegetarian, to find out if I had told her not to eat beef. The answer of course was no, but I couldn't help feeling somewhat annoyed. I had a public role in trying to find a way through this crisis, but my family had a right to privacy too.

In the midst of all this I went to Buckingham Palace to receive a knighthood from the Queen. I was also invited to Wembley by an old classmate, Professor Stuart Hillis, a cardiologist who was also the Scotland team doctor, for the Euro '96 game with England – astonishingly, the first time the two countries had ever played against each other in the finals of a major football competition. Sadly, for all Scots in the crowd

– and that included my son Andrew, who watched the game next to me with another old colleague, Dr Stuart Murray and his son – 15 June 1996 was the day Paul Gascoigne scored one of the most spectacular goals of his career as England beat Scotland 2–0.

* * *

The BSE/VCJD crisis would continue to occupy my attention for months to come. There would be many more meetings of SEAC, we would have to have another look at how the victims could be treated, how their families could be helped and recompensed, what the implications were for neurology, diagnostic and pathology services, how to make sure there was no possibility of any infected bovine material being used in vaccines, medicines or cosmetics, and much more. There would be an inquiry into the whole sad business and maybe I would even be scapegoated. I didn't – and still don't – think that I had done anything wrong, but being CMO at a time of a major health crisis can be a lonely and precarious job.

Right from the start of my medical training, I have always placed great store by the clinician's decision-making process. Underpinned by medical ethics, the general principles and priorities needed to provide a clear way through a crisis can become a lot clearer. In the case of BSE/VCJD these were:

- Base all actions on scientific evidence. In their absence, adopt the precautionary principle.

- Improve surveillance of both BSE and CJD, to ensure that any changes in their incidence are picked up as soon as possible.

- Direct all action at eliminating the disease in cattle, avoiding any risk of transmission to humans. When VCJD was identified in March 1996, the same principle applied to humans.

- Keep the public informed at all times about the disease, health risks and relevant research.

I have written quite a lot about risk.[8] It's a subject that has followed me around for practically all of my life in medicine. A woman who has had a mastectomy and is facing chemotherapy looks up at me and asks 'What are my chances, doctor?' A patient about to have a liver transplant asks about possibility of transfusion-transmissible infection. A journalist asks a CMO in, say, 1990 whether it's safe to eat beef. All of them, in different ways, are asking about risk. Because human beings are complicated organisms, and because our scientific knowledge so often falls short and we so often find ourselves dealing with the unknown, communicating risk is fraught with difficulty. It's a subject to which whole shelves of medical literature are devoted, and one which those three examples only illustrate in the most rudimentary way. Even in the case of breast cancer, one of the most intensively studied diseases in the western world, uncertainty still continued about best management, what to advise patients and, as we saw in the example of breast self-examination, what to include in national guidelines. In the case of transfusion-transmissible infections, our data is at least robust enough for patients in some countries to be given a mathematical assessment of the (negligible, one in a million) risks of acquiring, for example, malaria in a blood transfusion.

'Is beef safe?' is potentially a risky question to answer – even though when cows were dying of BSE, it was one that the CMO had to answer. The public were worried and they needed, quite rightly, to know. Yet look at what the answer to the question – asked, let's say, in 1990, when the link between BSE and the new disease of vCJD had not yet been established – should be and consider the pitfalls it has to avoid.

First of all, the answer has to be easily understood. It has to be clearly expressed, and has to reflect a culture of openness that itself is a necessary part of building up trust that any public health organisation requires. The answer, in other words, can't be avoided, procrastinated, or shrouded in obfuscating science-speak. So when Sir Donald, the CMO at the time was asked whether it was safe to eat beef, the press release quite correctly indicated that there was 'no scientific justification for not doing so'. In the clip they used on the TV news, his reply was edited down to a single sentence in which he said there was 'no risk' associated with eating beef. With BSE, according to our scientific knowledge at the time, that risk was remote, but it did exist. The CMO certainly knew that, but any such qualifications were, I presume, lost in the editing process.

When I took over as CMO in 1991, I commissioned a guide on just that topic for public health practitioners. Getting the words absolutely right is crucial – especially in a crisis like BSE/VCJD when nearly all of what the guide highlighted as the 'fright factors' that make risks more worrying to the public were in place. As all of those factors amplified existing fears about eating beef, when I was interviewed by the media about BSE, I always tried to provide an answer that reflected scientific realities rather than needlessly spread further alarm by also adducing unproven hypotheses and hunches.

As I have already mentioned, BSE had been on my radar since 1988 as a potential source of human disease. Yet only in 1996 did it turn out to be a provable source. Should I have mentioned this in public pronouncements even when there was no scientific evidence to back me up? Would that not have been irresponsible?

I cannot stress enough how important openness is in the field of public health. Not only does it confound the science-deniers and the conspiracy theorists ('It's all a government plot') but it is important in its own right. Provided patient confidentiality is protected, transparency is vital in dealing with risks to public health. I have always believed this and cannot think of any occasion where I didn't present relevant evidence during a health crisis as soon as it became available. But that doesn't mean that I feel I should tack on doubts, gut feelings, suppositions and suspicions to any health advice I gave when none of them had yet been cleared by science.

Translated into the clinical world, this would mean sharing such concerns with patients and families, but without clear evidence it would often be inappropriate. People may argue that patients or the public should make up their own minds about such things. But where does the doctor cross the line? When do you share a first suspicion of cancer with the patient, with all the alarm and fear such a conversation will bring in its wake? When you have a hunch that might soon be proved wrong? Really? Isn't it far better to wait until you have some scientific evidence, like a scan that not only shows a tumour but precisely where it is too? In hindsight – and just for once I'll allow myself some because I think it may well be relevant to future health crises – so much of the BSE crisis hinged on the accepted meaning of the word 'safe'. There still is, I feel, a degree of uncertainty about this – so much that, at least in the context of any discussion of public health, I think we should even consider banning the word altogether.

To me, to say 'beef is safe' does not mean 'eating beef is always going to be without risk'. This might seem like splitting hairs, but it is not. There is a fundamental difference between the two. If someone says that I am a safe driver, I do not take that to mean I will remain accident-free for the rest of my life, no more than if I tell you that it's safe to walk down the high street after dark I mean that there's no chance of you being mugged if you do. In both cases, all that I think is being meant is that the chance of me crashing my car or you being mugged is relatively small. There is always the possibility of someone driving on the wrong side of the road and hitting my car, just as there is of you meeting a psychopath down a dark alley.

Should we add those qualifications when giving any assessment of risk? Actually, I think we should. With hindsight, when I claimed that all of the existing scientific evidence suggested that there was no danger to human health in eating British beef, I should have added to the qualification 'as long as the regulations we have put in place are being enforced'. If I had added that, we might have avoided at least some of the media's misinterpretations.

One of the things I had realised as CMO was the divergence between scientists' perception of risk and the public's – and certainly the media's. A good example of this was the venous thrombosis scare that accompanied the launch of a new type of contraceptive pill in 1996. Its mortality rates of 1.5 per one million women per year, doubling to three per million women per year for the low-dose pill, led to plenty of scaremongering in the press, though that rate is still about the same as the risk of dying in a train crash and a lot less than the risk of being murdered (1:100,000). Few of us would live lives determined by such an unlikely event as murder and yet here so many of us were basing health decisions on something they were even less likely to face. Could we not, I wondered, find a new form of words that would allow us all to understand exactly what magnitude of risk we were talking about, the way we all roughly know the size of an earthquake from how high it registers on the Richter scale? I've tried hard to come up with something a bit like that, and to find out whether such a table of risk would work better as words (high, moderate, low, very low, minimal, negligible), or as illustrations, or as measured against population sizes (family, trees, village, small town etc). I don't think I've changed the world in this respect, although only the other day someone told me that the Australian National Blood Authority uses the 'Calman chart for explaining risk' to patients, so I haven't given up hope yet.[9]

All of that, and so much more, lay in the future back in March 1996, when the full extent of the BSE crisis became clear. The following month found me working on tests for HIV infection and wondering precisely why they, and radiological procedures, were not always 100 per cent reliable. In the middle of all of that, as I mentioned at the start of this chapter, I visited Jenner's House in the Gloucestershire village of Berkeley, where I paid my respects to the aforementioned Blossom (or at least her horn, which has pride of place in the museum to that great British benefactor of public health). Afterwards, I drove about 30 miles west towards the Cotswolds to see a long barrow near Avening in Gloucestershire. There are about 40 of these megalithic tombs in the county, and unlike most of them this wasn't built on top of a hill but in the middle of a field. It's way off any footpath and these days half-hidden by the copse of trees that has grown around it. Nothing special to see at all.

On top of it, there's a six-foot high stone, the last remnant of a chambered tomb atop the barrow. The stone has been there for some 6,000 years, and according to local legend, children used to be passed over it to cure them of infectious diseases. That's all I was trying to do too. If only, I couldn't help thinking, it was quite so easy.

CHAPTER 10

Make It So

FROM THE LAST couple of chapters, you could be forgiven for thinking that my job as CMO consisted of non-stop crisis management. In reality, though, the biggest improvements that can be made to a nation's health involve far less drama and take far more time. Real, lasting structural change can take months and years to bring about: strategies have to be set, a consensus built, reforms communicated, bureaucracies nudged, shifted and sometimes rearranged. In this chapter, I want to take a brief look at how, even within such a vast and complex organisation as the NHS, such changes can still be made to happen. Such writing might seem boring, but its purpose is to set out how a policy framework is developed and how it might be implemented. It may therefore be relevant to a wide range of interests.

Take, for example, improving the training of our hospital doctors. How can we ensure that they keep in touch with the latest developments in medicine and research? How can they best be trained on the job without reducing patient care? How can we ensure that standards of training aren't geographically patchy but consistently high? How can we measure that?

As you have probably already gathered, I place a high value on the importance of continuing medical education. For me, being a teacher is implicit in being a doctor – indeed, the etymology of the word itself (from the Latin docere, to teach) underlines that link. The two go hand in hand, and the high value doctors should place on medical education is reflected in the Hippocratic Oath itself, in which we all swore 'to hold him who taught me this art as equal to my parents'. But even though standards of medical education were generally good in the West of Scotland hospitals I visited when I was postgraduate medical dean at Glasgow University, I certainly realised that the training on offer at some hospitals wasn't as good as that which I had received myself.

As CMO England, I decided we needed to completely overhaul the way in which we trained hospital doctors. At its worst, this was haphazard, unstructured, and too little changed from 1968, when a Royal Commission had described it as 'chaotic'.[1] Doctors might attend occasional courses and conferences, but often not as part of a coherent training programme. In many cases, the training itself had no clear end-point, was sometimes duplicated, wasn't integrated with research and often lasted longer than necessary. Instead of continuous assessment, all the emphasis was on the 'big push' to pass external examinations. At a time when more women were going into medicine (in 1996 52 per cent of first year medical students were women) and there was greater demand for flexible training opportunities and part-time jobs, our old ways of doing things looked increasingly archaic.

The actual catalyst for reform was the European Commission's criticism of our specialist training accreditation. As far back as 1975, Brussels had been pushing for alignment between member states over minimum periods necessary for specialist training, but in the UK we had been dragging our feet. In July 1992 we decided to face up to the problem, but we also used the opportunity to look into the whole business of what we wanted from postgraduate medical education and address how any changes we made would affect career progression within the NHS. Although these reforms never caught the public's attention, within the world of specialist medical training they were transformational.

One of the potential weaknesses we identified was at the level of registrar and senior registrar. These were the grades doctors reached when they had already chosen their speciality and were on a career path towards becoming a consultant. The problem was that not only was there no fixed duration to these posts, but there was no structured training within them either. If, however, we created a new type of post, with a recommended training programme (including annual assessments) for each speciality, we could expect a host of benefits. There would be more medical expertise within our hospitals because they would have more consultants within them. This would in turn take some of the pressure off junior doctors, and might mean that registrars no longer became disillusioned working for years on end in the same job without the opportunity to make their way up the career ladder. Because of the new annual assessments, and because the new training courses encouraged individuals to undertake research projects, or at least to become more familiar with research methodology, we would have a clearer idea of doctors' abilities and they would be more aware of new treatments. The new training grade became known as the Calman Specialised Post, and the whole process became known as 'Calmanisation'. By March 1997, as many as 12,000 doctors within 53 specialities had signed up for it.

Put like that, this whole process of reform looks so easy, doesn't it? But let's unpick that process and see how what was, after all, the biggest change of its kind since the formation of the NHS came about.[2] First of all, a working party had to establish what needed to be done. That took from July 1992 to April 1993, when we published a detailed report on all aspects of the proposed reforms. And I do mean detailed: even boiled down to a précis, the report is still more than 100 pages long. But it had to be. Submissions from sixty organisations or individuals had to be taken. All the many and various institutions responsible for specialist training – the Royal Colleges, their faculties, and the postgraduate deans, along with all the regional general managers, directors of public health, private health insurers, health authorities, professional organisations and many, many more – had to be consulted and involved. Subgroups had to be set up to look in further detail at specialist training programmes, required standards for consultants, and how reforms would fit in with European legislation and medical training programmes.

As CMO, I chaired the working party, and set down a rigorous schedule for implementation of each of its recommendations. But just as consensus is vitally important in setting strategic aims, it was also important to keep a check on whether reforms were working out as we intended or whether there were any unforeseen problems. While the new reforms would of themselves add to hospital doctors' medical knowledge, we needed to ensure that this did not come at the expense of the experience they would need to cope with the undifferentiated emergency cases they would also encounter as consultants. That's why we welcomed a three-year comprehensive study into the effectiveness of the reforms from the Joint Centre for Education in Medicine. As the Prussian military theorist Carl von Clausewitz famously pointed out, 'no battle plan ever survives contact with the enemy', so it was important to check that Calmanisation worked in practice as well as in theory and survived contact with reality. In the end, we were satisfied that it did.

I only read Clausewitz's 1832 book *On War* years after I had finished being CMO. But when I did, I couldn't help thinking that quite a lot of what he wrote also applied to effecting change within a large organisation such as the NHS.

There are, he wrote, four things you must have in place if you are to stand a chance of victory. First of all, you need political will. Everyone needs to want the changes you envisage to happen. With the 1994 Calman Report, that condition was quite easily met. The Royal Colleges, the British Medical Association, and almost all other relevant bodies were generally supportive. The second requirement is for a clear strategy – in this case, something we had spent nine months developing by the time the working group delivered its report. The third necessity, according to Clausewitz, is to have people on the ground who have the skills and authority to make decisions. Here, our report scored highly, for we had the clear support of the postgraduate medical deans up and down the country, who were themselves responsible for training. The fourth and final factor in victory, he concluded, is having an effective supply line, which in an NHS context translates as having the financial resources, people, skills and buildings you need to effect your reform. Given the endless financial pressures on the NHS, this is often the hardest condition to fulfil. I keep a small note book with me at all times and notes of the projects in which I am involved. I check it regularly to assess progress, and if things are not going as planned, it is invariably due to one of these factors not being met. Indeed one can often do it before the project begins to assess its viability.

Let's keep the old Prussian military strategist in mind while we look at two more massive but slow-burn changes I helped to push through. The first of these is in the reorganisation of cancer care represented by another report with my name on it, although on this occasion, because I jointly chaired it with Dame Deirdre Hine, the CMO for Wales, it is known as the Calman/Hine Report (although I have sometimes heard it referred to as the Calvin Klein Report). It began one Monday morning in 1994 when I went up to Virginia Bottomley's office on the fourth floor. By then, she had been Secretary of State for two years, and that weekend she had held a surgery in her South West Surrey constituency at which one of her constituents had approached her to ask whether cancer services were better anywhere else in the country. 'Tell me, CMO,' she said, 'is it true that there's a postcode lottery in cancer?'[3] I had to agree that it was. 'Well, that can't be right,' she said. 'Can we do something about it?'

And that, in essence, is what it's like to be right at the epicentre of public health policy, and why I enjoyed my job as CMO so much. I have always been passionate about the NHS, and determined to do what I could to improve it. Asked by a journalist from *The Glasgow Herald*, just after I'd taken up the job, what challenge I most looked forward to being able to do something about, I singled out inequalities in health care provision: indeed, ever since we started Tak Tent we had always railed against such unfairness.[4] So when Virginia Bottomley asked if we could do something about inequalities in cancer service provision, as far as I was concerned, she was pushing at an open door.

As ever, the first thing to do was to set up a group of experts to look into the problem. Professional groups, health service managers, cancer charities, community groups and other organisations were all consulted. It was easy enough to agree on the need for high standards in cancer diagnosis, screening, patient-focused care, and that such high standards should apply uniformly across the country. Turning those ideals into reality was harder. This, too, was a complex report, involving the Royal Colleges, university departments, research groups, charities and health care professional bodies, and 300 different responses – collective and individual – were received; indeed, in the history of the NHS, it is reckoned to be the first such large-scale national plan of its kind.

What we found was a very mixed picture. Depressingly, apart from some fields such as testicular cancer (which accounts for 14 per cent of cancers in young men) in which the UK had a good track record, overall outcomes were generally worse in the UK than in Europe. Where there were proven levels of expertise in treating particular cancers, however, long-term survival rates increased by between 5–10 per cent. Noting this, we proposed that all patients with cancer be seen by specialists in their particular field rather than general surgeons, and that cancer centres should be established at designated district general hospitals. High-quality patient-centred communication and care – the importance of which had been proved in both Dame Deirdre's career as an expert in cancer screening as well as my own – would also be uniformly provided, as would early identification of cancers through screening and monitoring of effective treatment. Not only that, but we would work on the basis that treatment should always be a near as possible to where the patient lived.

Quite rightly, we were setting our standards high, but we were also being practical too, measuring what worked and improving outcomes. If we go back to Clausewitz's four points, there was a general agreement from cancer professionals on the points one and two (ie the changes we wanted to happen and the strategies we sought to bring it about). We were, however, weak on his third and fourth points: not only was there no clear delivery mechanism but the financial supply line was already stretched by the government's restructuring of the NHS to deliver the so-called internal market. Just at the time when co-ordinated regional planning could have helped, it seemed to be becoming less important. Despite that, a number of initiatives pushed the process forward. England's first national cancer plan in 2000 was largely based on Calman-Hine, but it also provided costings for the proposed changes, set specific objectives, and identified resources that could be used to achieve them – in essence, Clausewitz's points three and four. More than a decade on, a major study of how effective, or otherwise, Calman-Hine had been, argued that although change was variable and took longer than necessary, all the available evidence suggested that the policy was eventually successful and a worthwhile change.[5] The study's conclusion – that although the report was well thought out, sustained mechanisms for policy implementations are required if quality is to be improved – is completely fair.

The last of these major three health reforms came towards the end of my time as CMO, when I chaired a review that led to the creation of a one-stop phone helpline for hospital emergencies and – ultimately – NHS Direct. As ever, we assembled an expert committee, this time of people who provide emergency care, not only in the NHS itself but also the police, fire service, voluntary aid agencies and patient groups. A national helpline would, we concluded, help ensure that all emergencies were properly dealt with, including ones such as those caused by mental health, where many people didn't have a clear idea of whom they should turn to. And that mattered, because even though the 999 service enjoyed wide public confidence, 22 per cent of the calls it received did not result in patients being taken to hospital.

Blue lights, sirens and ambulances weren't always what was needed, we realised. In some cases, a phone line could be a new and helpful route into the emergency care service. Indeed, in some cases, such as providing information about what to do in the event of someone having a heart attack, it could literally be a lifeline. It also, come to that, loosely echoed an experiment we had done back in 1983 with Tak Tent in Glasgow, when we had established a separate 'cancer line' staffed by a doctor. Although this ran for one day only, and even then from just 9am to 6pm, we judged it a success, as in those nine hours we received 130 calls. As these were almost continuous, we estimated that between two and three times as many people had tried to get through but were unable to do so.[6]

Now, however, we were talking about providing a service on an altogether different scale, and something that ultimately led on to NHS Helpline 111, which to this day provides advice both over the phone (and now online) about when to go to A&E, when to go to an urgent care centre, and when to call 999. Three helpline pilot schemes staffed by nurses were set up in March 1998 in Lancashire, Northumbria and Milton Keynes, and the service was extended to the whole country within two years. By 2007 NHS Direct's website (which went live in December 1999) was receiving three million visits a month, which made it the largest service of its type in the world.

For guidance on overall health strategies, during my time as CMO we relied on two major policy documents. The first, The Health of the Nation, was produced in June 1991 under the Conservative government of John Major. Its objective was to lift attention beyond the day-to-day management of health problems and see what improvements we could make in the future. This involved setting out priorities and establishing targets in tackling problems such as coronary heart disease and stroke, cancers, mental illness, accidents, HIV/AIDS and sexual health. It was being produced and consulted upon just as I took up my post and became an important part of my own objectives. One of its themes was the need for people to take responsibility for improving their own health. As CMO, I echoed this by producing a leaflet in which I challenged everyone in the country to do something positive for the sake of their health. The first of these challenges was to take the stairs rather the lift. Within the Department of Health, we took this up so effectively that the stair carpet soon became so worn, it had to be replaced! In 1998, the second policy document, Our Healthier Nation, introduced by the new Labour Government, put a firmer emphasis on addressing health inequalities through measures such as establishing health action zones.[7]

And yet when I want to remind myself of my CMO years, the best guide to what we actually achieved isn't either the yellowing news clippings, the CMO's annual reports or those two national health strategy documents. Instead, it's a yellow ring-bound folder with, in two opposite diagonal corners, a drawing of electrons orbiting an atom, and a picture of a radio-telescope and three blue stars in the other two. And in the middle, in centred blue capitals, the title RAMBLINGS OF THE CMO: CAPTAINS (sic) LOG. It is, it's fair to say, not only very much a homemade production, but (and I mean this very kindly) one that has been made by someone without too much spare time on their hands. I should explain the title. In Star Trek I always liked the way in which Jean-Luc Picard managed the starship USS Enterprise, and in particular the two commands he would often use – 'Engage' and 'Make it so.' I found myself using the same terms in my regular emails to the staff, and when I left, these were bound into the said yellow ring-bound folder and presented to me.

Essentially, it's a weekly round-up of what I'd done during the previous week, and what I was planning to do in the next week or so, and the point of writing it was to keep the team abreast of what was going on. Sometimes I would request their help and expertise, but mostly I was reporting back from my various meetings and travels. As I turn its pages, I recall how all those big policy changes like improving training for hospital doctors came together one meeting at a time, and how they would still be going on at the same time as a health scare suddenly flashed on the horizon like a bolt of lightning. Nothing better captures the contiguousness of such wildly differently-paced issues, or shows more clearly just how many different issues were simultaneously bubbling away in both the background and the foreground.

Take MMR. In Ramblings of the CMO, it's easy to see the first stirrings of controversy, which came right out of the blue. In the early 1990s, immunisation coverage was one of our big success stories. GPs, working to a target-based payment scheme, were encouraging more and more children to be vaccinated. On top of that, new and more effective vaccines were being introduced, and as a result of just one of them, the commonest (Hib) form of meningitis had been effectively eliminated in 1992. In November 1994, seven million UK children were to be immunised against measles to head off an anticipated epidemic. When that happened, the UK would be on course to be the first industrialised country in the world to eliminate the disease. With just weeks to go before the school immunisation programme was due to begin, came the first stirrings of opposition. Because the manufacture of the rubella vaccine given alongside the measles jab involved cells that originated 30 years ago in the tissue of an aborted foetus, some Muslim and Roman Catholic faith leaders were calling for the vaccination programme to be boycotted. On 1 November, I had a meeting with them and reassured them that there were no foetal cells in the vaccine itself or, apart from the isolation of the original virus from an abortion on a woman with a rubella infection, were any involved in its current production. Thankfully, their doubts were allayed, and opposition to immunising their children largely vanished.

Three and a half years later, however, a small study in *The Lancet* purporting to show that the vaccine caused problems in the bowel, notably Crohn's disease, together with autistic spectrum disorders, was not so quickly dismissed and was taken up by the media.[8] After taking advice from the Joint Committee on Vaccination and Immunisation and the Committee on Safety of Medicines, I asked the Medical Research Council to convene a meeting to consider these issues at which those claiming there was such a link were given full opportunity to present their evidence. The MRC Expert Group concluded that as there was no substantive evidence of any link either with bowel disease or autism, there was no need to change immunisation policy. Sadly, even when disproved, scare stories live longer in the memory than positive ones, and even two decades later they still have a deleterious effect on public health.[9]

But my point about the *Ramblings of the CMO* is that it shows very clearly one thing that is always very hard to remember about the past, which is to say how many such issues were fizzing away at the same time, all stories with different deadlines, different levels of expertise required and different ways of being dealt with. We find it easy to remember one particular strand of a story, but what we tend to forget is precisely how other stories fitted in at the same time.

To show you what I mean, let's just take that same month – November, 1994. I'm not stacking the odds here; there were busier and more climactic months, and this one was relatively routine. I am picking it almost at random just to show the variety of the CMO's job. Two days after that productive meeting with faith leaders, for example, I was in Bonn for one of the six-monthly meetings of European CMOs. That particular meeting was a reminder that not everything on which we invested hope and money lived up to expectations, but back then the rest of Europe was still looking enviously at the NHS's IT project, then the biggest of its kind in the world, and my European counterparts were anxious to find out more about it from our briefing notes. There were many such meetings, and as well as keeping me informed about the various health reforms in other EU member countries, those trips added to my cultural hinterland: meeting in Rome, for example, we were treated to a private visit to the Sistine Chapel.

The international dimension of the job extended far beyond that, and Ramblings of the CMO often included accounts of the latest developments at Commonwealth ministerial meetings or European regional meetings of the World Health Organisation (WHO), whose Environment and Health Group I chaired. Working for the WHO not only put some of our health care problems into perspective but also allowed us to learn about new developments and possible new illnesses. In my time as CMO, HIV, Ebola, and influenza all figured prominently.

The UK has a seat on the Executive Board of WHO and I chaired this between 1998 and 1999. It was an exciting time, with change afoot in the organisation and opportunities to make a difference. One of my roles was to ensure that ministers in all relevant government departments were kept informed about anything which would affect the UK. I had the privilege of meeting the UK ambassadors in various countries, but notably the UK ambassador to the UN in Geneva. The WHO headquarters are in Geneva and I also took the opportunity to attend the Church of Scotland Sunday service in the Calvin Auditoire on several occasions.

From 1991 to 1999 I attended the World Health Assembly (WHA), the decision-making body of the WHO which brings together delegates from all its member states for an annual meeting in Geneva, which is attended by about 3,000 delegates from more than 150 countries. The assembly acts on an agenda set by the WHO's executive board, which also implements its decisions, submits proposals and can take emergency measures, if required, in association with the Director-General. A new Director-General, Gro Harlem Bruntland, a former three-term prime minister of Norway, was appointed in 1998 and this accelerated the changes needed and made the organisation more effective. The UK played an important role in effecting these changes and moving from one director-general to another.

Over my time in the WHO, I was involved in a number of important initiatives, including the elimination of smallpox, moves to wipe out polio, cut down smoking, roll back malaria and many others. Although strictly speaking unrelated to this work, I gained further insights into what it must be like to work as a doctor without many of the facilities we in the West take for granted when I was sent to Montserrat in September 1997 in the wake of a major volcanic eruption in which 19 people died. I was there with a small team to advise on the public health implications of the ash deposited and suggest solutions. The report I wrote was subsequently examined by a House of Commons Select Committee which set out some of the lessons learned.

It was a privilege to be part of WHO and see the passion and commitment for change and improving health all over the world. At the final WHA I attended in May 1999, I made a speech in which I quoted from an Ayrshire poet who put into words better than I ever could why we needed the World Health Organisation more than ever:

Then let us pray that come it may
As come it will for a' that
That Sense and Worth o'er a' the earth

Shall bear the gree an a' that
For a' that and a' that
It's comin' yet for a' that
That man to man the world o'er
Shall brithers be for a' that.

But let's get back to November 1994, and the same week as the European CMOs' meeting in Bonn and the meeting with the faith leaders over the rubella vaccine. In my report for that week, I noted that I was in the middle of a birthday dinner with my daughter on Sunday when the pager buzzed and I was invited onto ITN to talk about the MMR vaccination programme.

That Sunday night interruption was hardly atypical. The previous Saturday, my CMO logbook reminds me, had been largely given over to answering MMR queries from the media. These kinds of things had interrupted quite a few events Ann and I had been looking forward to – a 25th wedding anniversary dinner and an eagerly anticipated day out at the Chelsea Flower Show are just two that spring to mind, though there were plenty more. The demands of the media in London turned out to be of a completely different magnitude to anything I had experienced as CMO Scotland. On days heavy with health news, I would often find myself doing between seven and ten interviews on the same subject on the same day, moving round from studio to studio on what we referred to in the department as 'the Stations of the Cross'. Yet the media, I always realised, were doing a valuable job in informing the public about health and health care issues and in questioning medical experts and politicians, and a key part of my own job demanded that I be a good communicator too. Plenty of my colleagues would, I think, say that I was, but the more perceptive of them would realise that I sometimes worried that this was taking up too much time I could spend more productively on other matters.

But even though I did occasionally complain in the Captain's Log about such intrusions on my weekends, most other entries were far more celebratory. It is in the nature of the CMO's job that there are health centres to open, conference dinners to attend, speeches to be made honouring important figures and institutions (mine were invariably written in rhyming couplets). I'd sometimes slip in the odd bit of family news or (somewhat more rarely) refer to a Scottish sporting triumph or pass on news about the department's plans for the Christmas pantomime.

Not everything made it to the Captain's Log. On 7 December, 1994, Ann and I hosted a dinner for the Very Rev Dr James Simpson, then the Moderator of the Church of Scotland, and his wife. He had been in touch a short while beforehand suggesting that it would be rather nice to meet some Scots involved in the health field. This turned out to be quite easy to arrange. Nothing much seems to have changed in this regard since Tobias Smollet's 1748 novel *Roderick Random*, when the examiner at the College of Surgeons, on being told that Roderick had come down from Scotland, observed: 'We have scarce any other countrymen to examine you here. You Scotchmen have over spread us of late as the locusts did in Egypt.' This was, Dorothy L Sayers inferred in her novel *Five Red Herrings*, exactly the same state of affairs in 1931, when she has a Scot point out that 'all the big administrative posts in London were held by Scotsmen'. And it was certainly the same story in the Nineties too, because round our table we had (Sir) Allan Langlands, Chief Executive of the NHS, from Glasgow; Dr Sandy Macara and Dr Mac Armstrong, respectively the Chairman of Council and Secretary of the BMA, both Glasgow graduates; Sir Robert Kilpatrick, President of the General Medical Council, from Edinburgh; and Sir William Reid, the Health Service Commissioner, from Aberdeen. Unfortunately, Sir David Mason, from Glasgow, President of the General Dental Council, could not make it, but it still added up to a full house of Scots at the top of the health tree in England. And maybe that's why I didn't mention the fact in the Captain's Log. Sometimes it's not wise to boast.

Mentioning Sir Alan Langlands makes me think back to one of my proudest moments as CMO. On 3 July, 1998, the NHS was 50 years old, and a service of celebration was held at Westminster Abbey attended by Prince Charles and Prime Minister Tony Blair. There were some 1,800 health workers in the abbey, and the service began when 100 NHS staff carried a 20-yard-long banner showing images of the NHS across the years. Back then I felt about it as I did in 2018, when the NHS celebrated its 70th anniversary, and as no doubt I always will; that there is no clearer mark of a civilised society. The NHS has dealt with new treatments, new investigations, new diseases and an ageing population. In addition, it has improved the health of the nation and has an active programme of preventing illness. Of course it could do better, and all of its staff wish it to do so as well as to continue to provide care and compassion and treatment free for all at the point of need, and to carry on trying to make this country a healthier place in which to live.

As I walked down the aisle alongside Chief Nursing Officer Dame Yvonne Moores and Sir Alan Langlands, I don't think I have ever been prouder of the NHS in my life, and yet this was one of my last days officially working for it. Retirement at 60 was then mandatory for top civil service jobs, and even though that was still three years away, I wanted to carry on working. I wasn't quite sure what job I wanted to do next, but if I had seen an advert for a professorship in, say, public health policy, I would probably have applied for it. Being CMO was a high-pressure job that left very little room for family life, and a university professorship, probably in Scotland, would at least allow me to spend a lot more time with Ann. I owed her that, and I owed it to myself too.

While I was thinking along these lines, a friend mentioned that she had heard Durham University was looking for a vice-chancellor. Neither of us knew Durham, but we thought we would at least go there and have a look at the place. When we did, we liked it so much that when the headhunters at Saxton Bampfylde got in touch and asked whether I was interested in applying for the job, I said that I was, and went up for what turned out to be a successful interview. Every CMO there has ever been has retired when their period in office ended. But by the time of that Westminster Abbey service, I knew that in just a couple months' time there was, 264 miles to the north, a new challenge, a new job, and yet another wee adventure.

CHAPTER 11

The Durham Concerto

I LOVE ENGLAND'S cathedrals, and when criss-crossing the country as CMO, I always tried to squeeze in a visit to the nearest one if it was remotely possible. Impressive though so many are, none come close to matching Durham's massive patterned columns, ribbed high arches and vaulted ceiling. Look up at the light pouring through those high clerestory windows, imagine medieval masons cutting and placing those chevron-decorated stones in those monumental pillars, and even an atheist might feel awe. That feeling doesn't go away even when you go outside and look back at it: this is a building that dominates the landscape and indissolubly belongs to it. No wonder Bill Bryson, on the first of what turned out to be many visits, declared it to be 'the best cathedral on planet earth'. No wonder, too, that whenever anyone tries to work out Britain's favourite building, Durham's Anglo-Norman symphony in stone routinely tops the list.

The first time Ann and I saw it we were tourists, like most people making their way up to the cathedral's north door entrance. But within a year we were back, this time driving down from Glasgow ready to move into the vice-chancellor's residence. The final approach was easy enough: south down the A1, off west on the A690, the cathedral towers looming ever larger as we dropped down towards, and then across, the River Wear. We passed Old Elvet on our left, and I made a mental note: that's where I'd be heading the next day, to my office in the university administration building. Then up New Elvet, with the cathedral and what I would soon learn to call the Bailey on the right, turning right at the traffic lights and heading up towards what I would soon learn to call The Hill.

The Hill and the Bailey, that was how the colleges of Durham

University is divided up. The older ones, collectively known as the Bailey, clustering near the cathedral on the steep-sloping turn of the river at the historic heart of the city; the more recent ones, like Van Mildert and Grey College, about a mile away, up Church Street, in the suburban campus commonly known as the Hill. We were aiming for Grey College, because the map told us that was where we had to turn left, following the sign for the Botanic Garden. Hollingside, the vice-chancellor's residence, was right at the end of that road.[1] If I knew then what I know now, I'd have paid a lot more attention to the land on the left-hand side as we headed towards Grey College.

Why? Get to the end of the chapter and I'll tell you. But basically, it's one of those stories about how sometimes in life you pass somewhere and you don't realise it's going to have any enduring significance in your life. Just as, that first time Ann and I visited Durham to look at its Cathedral, neither of us realised that we would ever end up living in the city for nine years, that it would become a home, somewhere we cared about a great deal, and made so many friends that it was genuinely hard to leave.

**

For those nine years, my main job as Durham University's vice-chancellor was to try to maintain and enhance its reputation for educational and research excellence. The university was doing well, but I hoped to make it even better, and it was a key part of my mission to get the university moving back up to its rightful place at, or near, the top of the British university league tables. I had already identified key problems that needed to be addressed. We hadn't been raising enough money from our alumni, and some departments weren't delivering the kind of cutting-edge research we needed. Against that, student levels of satisfaction with their courses were reasonably high at both graduate and postgraduate level, so we didn't need to make too many changes there.

And still accentuating the positive, I wasn't intimidated by the challenge either. As postgraduate dean at Glasgow, I had gained some insight into the many and varied roles a vice-chancellor is expected to perform, and in the person of Sir William Kerr Fraser (the university's principal from 1988) and others before him seen how they could all be done flawlessly. The job of vice-chancellor requires a particularly disparate skillset, but it is one that mirrors the demands made on a CMO to a remarkable extent. True, I hadn't run a giant business, as some vice-chancellors had, but I had been the purse-holder for budgets bigger than most such businesses and had plenty of experience in managing change in a massive organisation. But the rest of the vice-chancellor's remit – speeches to a whole host of organisations, linking up with local and national politicians, being well-used to dealing with the TV, radio and print media, driving forward research, managing highly intelligent people, being on call for emergencies 24/7 – all of that was second nature to me by now. Even directing fundraising projects wasn't exactly alien territory.

Seasoned university dons reckon that it usually takes a full academic year before they can work out whether or not they have been landed with an efficient vice-chancellor or not. Only when they have seen vice-chancellors fulfil the whole range of tasks that the job entails, they argue, like how they cope at the matriculation ceremony in Durham Cathedral, or how well they chair their first meeting of the university Senate, can they begin to make any judgment on the newcomer's merits (or lack of them). And not even then. Those two events take place in the first week. The academics' assessment is far longer-lasting and more continuous than that, going on all the way through the university year. It continues through all the university council meetings, all the dinners with heads of the various colleges, all the way through to the graduation and honorary graduation ceremonies, and the first summer garden parties held at Hollingside. Each time, and at all times, a judgment of the vice-chancellor's effectiveness is being made. A university vice-chancellor is never fully off-duty.

I don't quite know whether it took Durham's academics a full year before they marked me down as an efficient vice-chancellor, and I hope it took a lot less than that. Certainly, I recognised what needed to be done fairly quickly: we changed how the university board operated, setting out a strategy to improve accountability and line management and deliver better learning and research in the biggest such re-organisation for 40 years. We identified what a great potential Durham had as a research university and set about trying to unlock it, by raising funds for teaching and research. We switched resources from relatively low-demand subjects to high-demand ones, bringing about more postgraduate research studentships in the process. Our sights needed to be raised for fundraising, so we raised them: by the time of Durham's 175th anniversary in 2007, the plan was, not only would all our academic investment plans be paying off but a new fundraising campaign would also have hit its £175 million target too.

It wasn't always easy. The Senate – the university's governing body for all academic matters – was often, to borrow a phrase from a retired vice-chancellor from Glasgow, 'a hotbed of cold feet'. Meetings could be noisy, sometimes even confrontational. A reorganisation that reduced the number of faculties from five to three also helped to make them less so, and corral the enormous collective intellectual power to better purpose, bringing people together in common cause rather than fighting fissiparous and often needless battles. I have often described my time as vice-chancellor as being like a director of an opera company. A university is full of prima donnas, a highly distinguished group of people who need constant support and to be told regularly just how good they are. The vice-chancellor's role is to provide the stage, the chorus, the props and the music, and hope that some of them sing the same opera.

By 2005, all that work as an academic opera director had started to pay off. That year, the *Sunday Times* awarded us their 'University of the Year' accolade. Underlining this, we also re-entered the list of the UK's top ten universities, a tribute to the outstanding teaching and research of the staff. This provided the university with an opportunity to celebrate its achievements, but also to thank the City of Durham, Stockton and the wider north-east for their support. That support, though, was mutual: the *Sunday Times* mentioned our students' engagement in the community as one of the reasons for giving us their top award, highlighting the work by Student Community Action and fundraising by students along with the collegiate environment, sports facilities and range of outside activities.

Academically, remaining a world-class university meant that we had to keep building on our strengths, even when it would have been far easier to argue that the new buildings and equipment or extra staff I was pressed to provide couldn't possibly be afforded. Durham at that time, for example, had – thanks to James Stirling's work on the behaviour of subatomic particles and his 22-year career at the university – one of the top physics departments in the world. We were delighted when Durham, not rivals with deeper collective pockets, secured funding for the new Ogden Centre for Fundamental Physics, and I did my best to ensure that we retained such competitive advantages because I knew full well how important it was us to have a number of subjects in which we unequivocally led the world.

Geography was another strong department, and here again we bent every sinew to ensure that it remained so. In 2000, at a time of financial stringency, we really couldn't, on any kind of quantitative assessment, justify creating six new lectureships in the subject. But, because I trusted the new head of department to deliver on his promises, we did just that. Two years later, that same department was awarded the very top external assessment rating possible.

A key part – arguably the most important – of the vice-chancellor's job is the appointment of senior staff. For a professorship, there would generally be three or four shortlisted applicants, each one of whom would be an expert in their chosen field. To have up to an hour with each was fascinating and I learned a lot about subjects I knew nothing about. Indeed, on one occasion I had such a good discussion that I followed it up afterwards to get further information – even though the individual was not appointed. The interviews were doubly valuable in that not only did they help me get to know who was joining the university, but the direction of their likely research.

One thing that was new to me about Durham was the colleges: I'd never been part of a collegiate university and after seeing how well the system worked at Durham, I rather wish I had. The colleges at Durham don't compete academically the way they do at Oxford and Cambridge, but they do in sport and much else. Each of them has its own proud history (going back in some cases to the founding of the university in 1832), and each student tends to have a strong loyalty to his or her college. They are, in other words, far more than glorified halls of residence, and are an integral part of the university's identity. Between the Bailey and the Hill, there were 12 colleges when we arrived, and as vice-chancellor I would have dinners at each of them in turn, which was an invaluable way of getting to know the students as well as the staff.

Outside Durham there were two more university colleges at the Queen's Campus (as it was renamed in 2002) 35 miles to the south at Stockton-on-Tees. Although this was originally intended to house the medical school, the campus now does invaluable work in providing foundation year courses that allow local (and now international) students the chance to go on to have a full university education. This is a cause particularly close to my heart. Many students, for a whole variety of reasons, leave school thinking that university is not for people like them. The foundation course showed them that, if they worked hard and passed their examinations, any and every Durham course would be open to them, apart from physics and mathematics. Yet to those students, as well as many others, I gave the warning: 'Don't let your degree get in the way of your education.' The words aren't mine, but I couldn't agree more with the sentiment: universities are not meant to be degree factories, but places where you can both have a good time and learn about the world.

Each year, at the campus, there was a diploma ceremony for the foundation year, and it was one of my favourite events in Durham's academic calendar. It was wonderful to see the range of students who had been successful. Many were women who had wanted to be teachers, and at the service it was great to meet them and their families, now that they had started on the first year of their degree courses at the university. In the first few years I met a medical school graduate and someone who had just gained a PhD. I was proud to be part of such an imaginative rethinking of the university's role.

When I first joined, the degree ceremonies in Durham were held in the hall of University College, or Castle as it is usually known because it is mainly housed in Durham Castle and hence is the one of oldest university buildings in the world (construction on the castle began in 1072, 13 years before work began on the cathedral). But the hall had now become too small for our purposes, so into the cathedral we went. And what better place could there possibly be? The ceremony took place only a hundred yards or so from the tomb of a man the great medieval historian Sir Richard Southern hailed as 'first major intellect produced by the Germanic peoples of northern Europe', reckoned by many to be 'the father of English history' and by Dante to be dancing in heaven with the other great theologians. The Venerable

Bede had lain there since the cathedral was built all those years ago. Perhaps this was another reason I liked Durham cathedral so much: here learning, and veneration for learning, was in with the bricks.

In the meanwhile, those fresh-faced graduates would have also encountered another amazing man. Sir Peter Ustinov, who was then Durham's chancellor, could speak ten languages, give a wise, wit-drenched speech at the drop of a hat and was charm personified. When we moved our graduation ceremonies from the castle to the cathedral, he wondered whether he would be able tell jokes in such a deeply spiritual setting, but he seemed to get away with it. Ann and I adored his company when he came to stay with us at Hollingside, where he sometimes tested out on us the jokes with which he would later regale an audience.

Ann made sure that Hollingside played an increasingly important part in the social life, not only of the university but of the whole sur-rounding area. She had been given carte blanche to redecorate the whole building after it had been cleared of asbestos, and took advan-tage of the building works to widen the doors between two of the four huge downstairs rooms. Before, the narrowness of both the doors and the corridor between them made receptions rather awkward; the renovations transformed the house into a place where people could gather together a lot more easily. A downstairs catering kitchen and a dining room that could, as for our Christmas dinner get-togethers, cater for three dozen guests, completed the house's transformation. The downstairs would, we decided, be effectively given over to the university functions; we, along with our dog Mungo, would mainly live upstairs. Hollingside became not only a hub of academic social life but – filling a role that had perhaps been somewhat neglected – helped to bring town and gown closer together, as well as building up links with important people in the region. Garden parties, luncheons and dinners were a regular occurrence, as were functions for college staff and students. I even composed a special grace for such events:

We, who in the footsteps of Cuthbert and Bede
Thank you for this Fellowship and all the food we need
For the Cathedral, this City and the wider north-east
So we think of others, and not least

Of those whose needs are greatest, give them the happiness they seek
And for our special guests this evening, 'lang may their lum reek!'

This latter phrase confused some people in the north-east but it refers
to having a nice warm fire at home!

The role of the vice-chancellor's partner is often forgotten, but Ann
was crucial in helping me establish the way non-academic aspects of
the university were run, from drawing up menus for dinners to welcoming guests, ensuring visitors were seated in the correct place for
graduation ceremonies and looking after our visiting chancellors. At
the same as doing this she was chairing the County Durham and Dar-
lington Primary Care Trust, a major NHS operation. I could not have
done it without her help.

My own speeches may not have been as effortlessly witty as Sir
Peter's but there were certainly a lot of them. I have a folder full of
them all written on small cards and generously sprinkled with jokes.
I began a file of jokes and quotations at that time for such occasions,
and it is still worth a look! Some of those speeches worked better
than others. One I remember in particular was at the Castle, when the
guest of honour was the Lord Chancellor, Baron Irvine of Lairg. As I
finished the first page of my speech of welcome, I placed it on the table
and carried on with the second. I was halfway through that when I
realised that the discarded sheet had caught fire from a nearby candle
and was burning away. Fortunately, the fire was quickly extinguished
before the evening became memorable for all the wrong reasons.

Until I looked though the diary I had forgotten how many of those
speeches were delivered to foreign audiences. During my time in Durham I visited Japan, Sri Lanka, the USA, Barbados, Thailand, New
Zealand, Australia, Jordan and India. Meanwhile, back in Durham,
I made a few more as a Deputy Lieutenant of the county. At the university itself, there were a few more big changes in store. One of the
most exciting was the establishment in 2006 of an Institute of Advanced Studies (IAS). This was a flagship project linked to the 175th
anniversary, and reaffirmed the value of ideas and the public role of
universities. The IAS aimed to cultivate thinking on ideas that might
change the world, through unconstrained dialogue between disciplines as well as interaction between scholars, intellectuals, and public

figures from a wide variety of backgrounds and countries. Its focal point was a programme of work based on an annual theme linked to a fellowship programme, and each year at least 20 highly creative individuals were invited to spend up to three months at the institute's centre. We chose Cosin's Hall, a beautiful Georgian building on Palace Green that had been a student hall of residence when Durham started life as a university for this purpose. During their stay there, the IAS Fellows also engaged with the colleges, departments, the students and the community through conferences, seminars and workshops. The inaugural theme was 'The Legacy of Charles Darwin' and this attracted a wide range of interests and participants. Another venture the IAS spawned was *Thinking About Almost Everything*, a book launched in 2009 and partly inspired by our new chancellor Bill Bryson's book *A Short History of Almost Everything*. The IAS continues to grow and provide a forum for debate and discussion on topics of wide interest.

Even closer to my heart was the creation of the Centre for the Art and Humanities in Health and Medicine in Durham in 2000. Its first director was Dr Jane MacNaughton, who happened to be a student in Glasgow in the 1980s when Professor Robin Downie and I began using literature to illustrate ethical issues in medicine. The centre was set up to examine the growing evidence base that the arts and humanities have a role to play in health and health care. It acts as a resource for policy-makers as well as carrying out research and evaluation, and to develop the discipline of the medical humanities. It, too, has gone from strength to strength.

The two books I was writing in Durham were on, if not exactly similar then at least parallel lines to the topics being explored at the new centre. But both *Storytelling, Humour and Learning in Medicine*, and *A History of Medical Education* kept me in the library for many hours, at least the students and academics seeing me there probably realised that we were all on the same side. I also continued to do some teaching in the fields of history, law, anthropology and medicine and that might have boosted my credibility a bit too. Thinking about *A History of Medical Education* reminds me of Mungo, the flatcoat retriever we bought just as we moved into Hollingside and named after Glasgow's patron saint, because he also appears on the book's inside cover.[1] He is there too in a superb portrait of me the university commissioned from Anne Mackintosh in 2005. At first, she said this might be difficult, but I was able to persuade her, and the resulting portrait has me in full vice-chancellor's dress, with Mungo sitting at my feet and looking up proudly but inquisitively. My children have on occasion noted that while I included a picture of Mungo on that book jacket, I didn't include one of them! The portrait was based on a photo taken (with, I hasten to add, the Dean's permission) inside Durham cathedral, which is yet another reason that building is embedded so firmly in my affections.

Mungo was helpful in other ways. Hollingside was in the Botanic Gardens and a wonderful place to have events and parties. When these were taking place, Mungo was kept upstairs in the house, but when it was time for visitors to go, he was released and joined the crowds. This was always a very efficient, but still polite, way of signalling that it was time for guests to go home, and Mungo became well known in the university and the city as guests said goodbye to him as they left.

And so to 2007, the year we had been looking forward to for so long. We lost the wonderful Sir Peter Ustinov in 2004, but by the following year we had a new chancellor, Bill Bryson: my appointment, and, I have to say, an inspired one. In *Notes from a Small Island* he had described how he got off the train at Durham on a whim, never having heard of the place other than some mention of its cathedral, only to find himself in the middle of a 'perfect little city'. His affection for Durham never dimmed, and he has written that his time as chancellor was the happiest of his life. Speaking on behalf of the university, I can say that the feeling was mutual. Sir Peter was a hard act to follow, but Bill managed to do so. The fact that the new university library is named after him is a tribute to how well he did the job.

For our 2007 celebrations, the colleges had mobilised their alumni as never before, and the fundraising target of £175 million had been surpassed with many millions to spare. We decided to commission a piece of music from the composer, Deep Purple co-founder and keyboard player Jon Lord and thus The Durham Concerto was born. Based around a day in the life of Durham, it is in six movements, from dawn breaking over the cathedral until the evening, when the students singing *Gaudeamus Igitur* (my suggestion) bump into a band at the

miners' gala. The world première took place on 20 October 2007 at
– where else? – Durham Cathedral, with the Royal Liverpool Philhar-
monic Orchestra joined by Lord himself on the Hammond organ and
Kathryn Tickell on the Northumbrian pipes and it was an absolute
triumph. Since then, it has been performed at least 40 times around
the world.

I could very easily end the Durham chapter of life there, as I was
elected chancellor of Glasgow University on 26 January 2006, although I remained vice-chancellor at Durham until 2007. By the time
I left, there were two new colleges – Ustinov (for postgraduates) and
Josephine Butler (named after the Victorian women's campaigner) –
at what I would have to learn to call The Mound, which was further
up the Hill, past Grey College. Overall, the university was back to its
old, academically successful ways. Ann and I (and Mungo) had been
happy there, and we had learnt enough about the north-east of England to concur with our new friend Bill Bryson that its people were
indeed the friendliest in the country. And The Durham Concerto was
indeed, some kind of apogee, a natural musical high, a fitting note on
which to bow out. So why won't I?

The reason is that I still haven't told you something I promised,
at the start of the chapter, that I would. If you remember, we were
driving up South Road – in the very direction of Ustinov, Josephine
Butler, John Snow and Stephenson Colleges, all of which, back then,
were still to come into being. At the city end of South Road, there
were similar blank spaces on the map that today have been filled by
buildings a new generation of students has come to know and love. If,
back in 1998, Ann and I had looked to our left at the traffic lights at
which the road begins, we wouldn't have seen the huge glass frontage
of the Palatinate Centre, which now not only houses the Law School
but also the university's administrative buildings and student support
services. No Institute of Hazard, Risk and Resilience at the bottom of
the hill, no new School of Geography, no Bill Bryson Library either.
All those buildings would come into being in the couple of decades
after Ann and I headed up South Road on our way to Hollingside
on our first day in Durham. The site they were built on was a large,
empty field turning into a forested slope as it rose away from the city.
There was nothing there to look at, so the land which then became

Durham's Science Centre would have just flashed by in a couple of seconds as we drove along.

And yet now, on this land, in the middle of the Science Centre, with the Biophysical Sciences Institute on one side and the Department of Computer Science on the other, there's a building that means almost as much to me as any in Durham, even though it was built after we left. The Calman Learning Centre is the main lecture theatre complex for the Science Centre. I was particularly honoured that they named it after me, and I liked the title, as learning is at the heart of the university, and indeed my life, and I was honoured to be asked back to open it in April 2008, when we returned to the campus and met old friends. The lecture theatres in the building are named after some Durham greats – Professors Barrett, Cramp, Wade and Sir Arnold Wolfendale – and it was a privilege to be associated with their reputations. It has been so built that lectures shown in one main theatre, if over-full, can be shown live in two slightly smaller theatres – catering at most to an audience of over 1,000. That, and the two cafes within it, means that the building could also be used to host research conferences, which gives it added functionality in the fast-changing world of universities.

Most of the time, I imagine, it will be where undergraduates start making their first steps on their own journeys of learning. To all of them, and particularly the ones whose schooling wasn't the easiest, or who have triumphed over adversity and taken a second chance on the academic life via the foundation year programme, the chap whose portrait hangs above the main door of the building (that man in the red gown in Durham Cathedral with a beautiful black dog called Mungo at his feet) sends his very best wishes.

CHAPTER 12

Me and My Mace

MUSIC MAKES ME cry easily, especially when the lyrics are laced with meaning, and especially when the service that they are both part of is too. Call me predictable, but the Irish Blessing sung by the choir at the end of the Commemoration Day service in Glasgow University's Bute Hall gets me every time. Commemoration Day, I should explain, is one of the most important days in the Glasgow University calendar. It's the service at which we bestow our honorary degrees, when the Lord Provost and other leading lights of the city come along to join us, when all the academic staff will gather in their full academic gowns, and when we honour our founders and benefactors.

I say 'we' for a couple of reasons. First, because Glasgow University is the one place at which I have studied for all of my four degrees, and the Victorian Gothic splendour of Bute Hall is where I have been awarded them. And secondly, because for the last 13 years I have been the university's chancellor.

So when, at the end of the Commemoration Day service the choir sings out,

> May the sun shine warm upon your face;
> the rains fall soft upon your fields
> and until we meet again,
> may God hold you in the palm of His hand

and the chaplain gives the blessing, it is one of those ultra-rare moments of predictable joy. As I climb down, damp-eyed, from the podium, usually I am still marvelling at the achievements we have all just heard listed about our honorary graduates. Then, because being chancellor means that you also get to choose the music the university organist plays for the ceremony, you can find yourself leading the platform party out of the hall to a tune you really like: in 2018, when I had just awarded my daughter Susan an honorary doctorate, we all marched off to the theme from *Star Wars*.[1] To all of this, add spectacularly unGlaswegian weather – and you often can, because Commemoration Day takes place around midsummer – end-of-term joie de vivre, bagpipes, whisky, a colourful procession round the East Quad, and all with the prospect of an enjoyable lunch to come, and even the most dismal pessimist in the world might be won over.

It was at such a ceremony on 21 June 2006 that I was installed as chancellor. I was still vice-chancellor at Durham in January that year when I won the election for the chancellorship of Glasgow against Sir Neil MacCormick.[2] My installation ceremony began in the university chapel. Of course I knew the place well, and I knew what the service consisted of too, and how to some members of the congregation the recitation of names of the university's benefactors might seem tediously long. But not to me. Because that rollcall of names was more than just a list, it was an idea of a university made flesh in each successive generation, all the way back to 1451, when a Pope had agreed with a request from one of his more distant bishoprics, that there should indeed be a university in Glasgow, and that it should have all the rights and freedoms enjoyed by the one at Bologna, the oldest in Christendom. So the silver thread began, with the charter sent from Pope Nicholas V to Scotland's King James II, and it is a benefactors' list on which rivalries and hatreds drop away and all that remains is support for learning; a list where Charles I can be mentioned right next to Oliver Cromwell and the city's magistrates are thanked for preserving the university 'in times of civil war and commotion'; and on it goes, from the Marquess of Montrose to Andrew Carnegie, from William Hunter to the Wellcome Trust. All benefactors 'by whose liberality this college and university has maintained the studies of godliness and sound learning'.

In all that time, there have been 41 others chancellors of Glasgow University, each serving an average of more than 13 years – longer than most popes, presidents and prime ministers. For the first century of the university's existence, the chancellors were all bishops or archbishops, as Pope Nicholas had originally intended. In the whole of the 18th century, by which time Commemoration Day (which began in 1690) was already up and running, there were just four chancellors; there were only five in the 19th. Meanwhile, the idea of what the university should be was constantly changing, indeed it was physically moving from one part of the city to another, being added to and built on, and the people who had helped to do that, who had been its ambassadors and lead office-holders were celebrated in the very Memorial Chapel in which, on that June morning in 2006, my family and I were gathered, along with honorary graduates and representatives from 11 other universities.

Soon, I would become part of that long tradition myself. Affixed on the walls above the choir stalls were the coats of arms of all those 41 other chancellors, all the way back to Bishop Turnbull, to whom Pope Nicholas wrote the document that brought the university into being. There was a space at the end nearest to the congregation where my coat of arms would one day go. I never needed one before, but to take my place in the ranks of Glasgow's chancellors I needed that, and a motto too. Cum Scientia Succurro ('through knowledge I help others') made sense for the latter, but what symbols should I choose for my life? In the end, I picked four: a tree (standing for Glasgow) at the bottom of the shield, a golden arrow (a much more ancient symbol of medicine than the more conventional intertwined snakes of the Caduceus) on a blue band above it, and on top of both an open book and a wheatsheaf (the symbol of the Incorporation of Bakers in Glasgow, of which I am a member). There it is in one picture: the story of my life.[3] If you ever go to the Memorial Chapel and find the shield, look on the pew in front of it and you'll find a carved wooden figure of a monkey next to a palm tree. No, I don't know what it's doing there either.

For the second part of the service – the actual installation – we walked round to the Bute Hall, which was packed with all the leading figures in the university, honorary graduates and civic dignitaries. In my speech, I tried to explain what the university meant to me. Because I have spent so much of my working life in universities, I would like to expand on those thoughts later on in this chapter, but that day I went right back to the start of that silver thread, to what Pope Nicholas had in mind when he first imagined a university in the west of

Scotland. He expressed it differently, but he, like me, believed in the power of learning, that it was a 'blessing ... which shows him the way to live well and happily, and by the preciousness thereof makes the man of learning far to surpass the unlearned, and opens the door for him clearly to understand the mysteries of the universe'.

Like Cardinal Newman in *The Idea of a University*, Pope Nicholas stressed importance of providing teaching on a wide range of subjects and urged that 'every lawful faculty should be set up... where the simple [are] instructed, equity in judgement upheld, reason flourish, the minds of men illuminated, and their understanding enlightened'. The Pope also emphasised that the university should be not just for Glasgow, but for Scotland 'and the regions lying about', by which I suppose he meant England. Again, spot-on; again, truths about education that have stood the test of time. Back in the 21st century, I went on to talk about the role the university could play in establishing a cultural quarter in the West End of Glasgow, and how we could strengthen and deepen our links with the city, widen participation, and develop new models for research.

Before I began my speech, I had been helped into my chancellor's robes – heavily gold-embroidered black gown and gold-tasselled mortarboard. At that moment, I became chancellor, so this was my first service in the role. At its end, after the red-robed choir up in the balcony sang the Irish Blessing and the organ swelled, I followed the beadle – or bedellus to use the proper Latin – and his mace as we went out of the hall. And as I write this, I've just thought of another reason why Commemoration Day matters. It's the tiniest of details, yet it points to something so big that it is hard to express. If you look up at the chandeliers in Bute Hall, you will notice that the lights on them are not arranged horizontally, as one would normally expect. Instead, they are six-foot high columns of lights on five levels, tapering towards the top, like a narrower and longer version of the papal tiara. What they are actually meant to copy is the bedellus's silver mace, which the university commissioned back in 1460. The dangerous end of the mace – although as far as I know it's never been swung in anger, though it did disappear for 30 years during the Reformation – is a hexagonal three-story tower made of gold and enamel. History, in other words, is all around us, sometimes in small details we might not know about – Victorian chandeliers and medieval maces commissioned, bequests made, books read, studies finished, degrees obtained. And on Commemoration Day, when almost everyone in Bute Hall is dressed, rather timelessly, in academic gowns, you can sometimes catch a glimpse of our own small place in time too, and it is both humbling and oddly comforting.

There is another reason that Bute Hall is, for me, a place of great happiness: it is where they hold the university's graduation ceremonies. And when I look down from the chancellor's chair at all those bright young faces of students about to receive their degrees, I remember what it was like to be like them, when all the options in life were as wide open as they ever could be. I think back to how I felt on 6 July 1967 when, along with about 140 colleagues, I had sworn the Hippocratic oath in the hall next door[4] and we had all set out into the world to become doctors.[5]

As part of graduation day, I get to say a few words, and I always try to tailor them to whatever subject the people in front of me have graduated in. One year, for graduates in veterinary medicine and surgery, I read out a poem I'd written about Mungo, the flatcoat retriever we had bought in Durham and named to remind us of Glasgow:

The kitchen was the first place
Dog biscuits, other food, dishes and toys
Littered debris and smelly towels
Floor swept and washed and black hair removed
The long hall took longer
The hoovering took the time
And picking up the toys outside the bathroom
Where he drank and lay, needing special attention
Lounge and dining room took little time
But the den where he slept and
Beside our bed where he lay
Will need proper cleaning.
It was the study which hit me
My own room where he lay beside me
And I stroked his handsome head
That I found it, between the shredder and the bookcase

It was… his duck
Chewed, yellow feet torn off
Holes in it and ragged
But it was his
He brought it to the door when we came in
He took it to the kennels
He laid his head on it
And we played with it, pulling till it ripped even more
Unlike the others, I couldn't throw it out
Discard it for ever
I will keep it in a special place
In Brodick where he loved the sea
I knew where he would be on Brodick
He swam for hours no matter the temperature or the wind
Swimming with the swans and seals
Alive and happy
As I will remember him, and his duck

Whatever the subject, though, I'd express what I genuinely hoped, that the students would keep up their link with Glasgow University, that they would carry on learning, and that their lives would be happy and intellectually fulfilled. And then the choir would sing the Irish Blessing and I'd get moist around the eyes again and the organ would peal out its own aural blessing, and we would process out of the hall, led by the beadle and his mace. And if you can find a more intoxicating mixture of hope and knowledge and happiness than that which as I – and, I hope, they – feel as we leave the hall, go down the stairs to meet the piper, and then follow him round the East Quad to drinks in the Cloisters, with its wonderful views over the city – if you find that anywhere, I'd like to hear about it.

It's not as though I've forgotten what it's like to be on the receiving end of a graduation ceremony too. On 27 June 2013, I was awarded an MLitt in the subject of Scottish Literature and Medicine – the first chancellor since 1451 to be awarded a proper degree while in post! It was fascinating being a student again, and I was delighted to thank Professor Gerry Carruthers Professor Kirsteen McCue for all their help. For the ceremony, I led the procession into the hall as usual, took a seat below the vice-chancellor, Sir Anton Muscatelli, and award-ed two honorary degrees.[6] Then I moved to the side, changed my gown and when my name was called, came forward to have the de-gree awarded by the vice-chancellor, and returned with the rest of the graduates to sit with them. At the end of the ceremony I processed out with my fellow graduates to the *Star Wars* theme.[7]

After so many years at Glasgow University, my love of the place is multi-layered. I follow its expansion with interest and excitement: the one billion pound project currently constructing a new business school, learning hub and research centre on the site of the Western Infirmary is probably the biggest of its kind in Scotland. But I have also learnt to treasure the small details of university life as well as its big dreams. I'll give you just one example of what I mean, though I can think of hundreds. I have already mentioned the Memorial Chapel, and it was indeed built to honour the memory of the 755 Glasgow University graduates who died in the First World War (as well as those who died in subsequent ones). Yet at Glasgow we take that commemoration one step further. On the individual anniversaries of their deaths, these graduates are also mentioned at a small service at the chapel and a small named cross and a poppy is placed that day in the memorial garden.

A university is, after all, a place where small threads of knowledge and experience are woven into something more, and in my case that applies to Glasgow University itself. If I didn't feel this, I would probably give up the job right now; for someone with an arthritic right hand, 200 handshakes in the course of a single ceremony can be mildly painful. And you'd never think it, but the embroidery on the gown is so heavy that it actually ripped the sleeve of three of my suit jackets before I came up with an improvised solution and added another protective cloth layer.

Although as chancellor I am not involved in the day-to-day work of the university, there are some areas in which my role widens beyond the ambassadorial. One of these is in relation to the Hunterian, Scotland's oldest public museum. This was founded with a munificent gift from William Hunter, who was born in East Kilbride and trained in Glasgow. He moved to London, where he, along with his brother John (a surgeon), became one of the most successful physicians in the country. Hunter's collection, which ranges from art to medicine, is world-class, but a big issue for the museum was how best to display it and use it to encourage research and teaching. This has now been successfully achieved with a series of Master's programmes in curatorial practice. The collection itself has begun to move to a new location, the Kelvin Hall, close to both the university and the Kelvingrove Museum, allowing a real opportunity to work together. In addition, the National Library of Scotland's Moving Image Archive has also moved to that location so further partnerships can be built.

The second example of a project I have been involved in, is the University Settlement, a charity founded by pioneering women students in 1897 with the aim of supporting people in the poorer areas of Glasgow. They 'settled' in such places and provided the poor with practical support in different ways. Helped by a small fund, today's students mirror that work with projects they work on for charities in their summer vacation. When term starts again, the students present their work to a university audience together with representatives from the charities. These are inspirational events, and are firmly based on the original principles of the Settlement.

The chancellor's ambassadorial role is a fulfilling one in its own right, and it is a privilege to meet alumni groups across the country and beyond, bringing them up to date with how well the university is performing. I often attend special services in the university chapel, as well as the annual service in Glasgow Cathedral (where the university was founded) and I have even represented the university at Buckingham Palace, as I did for an event during the Queen's Diamond Jubilee.

Quite apart from being chancellor, of course, I have worked in universities as a student, lecturer, professor, dean, and vice-chancellor. It would be odd if, over the years, I hadn't thought about how they can help to create new knowledge, transmit it more efficiently to the world and foster better conditions for research. So what, in short, should the dynamic 21st century university aim to be? I should give an immediate health warning: there is not one single ideal of what a university should be that would fit all needs, and there never has been. Universities are dynamic organisations which change with time and are constantly developing and responding to outside and inside pressures. They will need to continue to do so.

When it first started life in 1451, for example, the University of Glasgow had four regents who taught arts, theology, medicine and civil law. In practice, arts dominated. By the 18th century, however, the range of subjects studied had widened considerably to include Greek, mathematics, logic and rhetoric, natural philosophy, divinity, Hebrew and Semitic languages, anatomy, botany, and astronomy. In the 21st century that expansion has continued apace, as one would expect from a university with over 26,000 students and a teaching budget of over one billion pounds.

Dictionary definitions of 'university' quite rightly put the emphasis on people, not buildings. It is the community of learning that matters, not bricks and mortar. And when we look at the differences between a school or a further education college, and a university, this is equally apparent. All three are places where one might go to learn, but at the university the teachers are also scholars and at the leading edge of research in their subject. This is an essential difference and allows the unique nature of a university to be characterised. It is not just a place of learning, it is more than that. That extra is its essence, its uniqueness, its scholarship and research in a community bound by tradition, the desire to know more and to use that knowledge for the benefit of others.

Universities are – or should be – exciting places to be, filled with creative minds tackling new ideas. And because they are living institutions, they are constantly changing and developing, even while they remain an organic whole. A university is always far more than a series of unrelated schools which just happen to be located on the same site. To be truly effective it requires a wide range of students, with a good mix of genders and of social and racial backgrounds, and an equally wide range of subjects taught. But what else is needed for the truly 21st century university?

The first thing I'd look for is new and original thinking. This is sometimes described as 'blue sky' thinking; intellectual work which may have no immediate practical outcome, but which provides a basis for radical changes in concepts and ideas. It is not confined only to the sciences, but covers all disciplines, and is what puts the 'higher' into higher education. Technology transfer and innovation is vital in the generation of new businesses, and can transform the economy of a region, though they are often high-risk ventures and the number of people employed may be limited. But there's far more to a successful society than that, and the university should also provide social, economic and cultural innovations too. This includes the arts, education and activities including sports and leisure. Universities have a major role in supporting the very fabric of society, integrating with local cultural organisations such as museums, art galleries and botanic gardens.

All societies have disadvantaged groups and universities have a role in providing the thinking and new ideas which might help to transform their lives. Providing more routes into education would be a good way of doing this. The traditional way has been via appropriate levels of knowledge and skill gained in school. But we need a wider vision, particularly to encourage those from disadvantaged backgrounds to gain entry. To see young people, learn, grow and develop, and watch their subsequent progress, is a very powerful part of the academic role. As the medieval Jewish polymath Maimonides wrote:

> Much wisdom have I learned from my masters, more from my friends, but most from my pupils. Even a small twig kindles a great fire, so a little pupil stimulates the rabbi and there goes out from his questions marvellous wisdom.

In this context, a distinction needs to be made between education and training. Training is directed towards the acquisition of specific skills. Education is a broader process and deals with more generic issues. One of my favourite mottos is 'To be trained is to arrive, to be educated is to continue to travel' and a good 21st century university education might involve taking that literally as well as metaphorically, as students search out the best 'knowledge magnets' for their purposes.

To an extent, they always have. Take studying medicine. In medieval times, the place to go was Salerno in Italy, then Bologna, Padua, and Montpellier. By the 18th century the focus of study had moved to Leyden and Edinburgh, then in the 19th century, Berlin, Paris and the universities of the United States of America, and so on into our own age. Medical students have travelled to the best places to study and still do. The 21st century university should certainly aspire to fulfil the World Health Organisation's concept of the 'healthy university' in which the health of staff and students is a top priority. This goes a long way beyond just giving advice on diet, exercise, drugs and alcohol, and extends to proper facilities and resources for both mental and physical health and ensuring that individuals with problems can be identified and support offered.

After they leave the university, alumni matter more than ever before. The university and the colleges need to keep in touch, by sending information about new developments and possible postgraduate opportunities. Similarly, the student will wish to let the university know of his or her progress (staff have great pride in knowing how well people do) and if possible, giving back some expertise or resources to the university. This is a special partnership and we need to do more to support it. Alumni can be of great use to the university and they are usually more than happy to support its initiatives. Lifelong learning is also vital to the 21st century university. Graduates should be kept informed about new courses, degrees, conferences and seminars, but the university should never lose sight of its outreach function too. Both need different strategies and approaches.

To achieve its aims, the 21st century university needs a clear strategy, and while broad vision statements set the tone, it is the action plan which will deliver the outcome. This also needs to be linked to a timescale, and methods of measuring its implementation that will allow problems to be identified early on and changes in direction made before difficulties arise. Setting targets gives a sense of direction, purpose and priorities, and the kinds of resources required to achieve them.

The 21st century university should, however, make sure that it always retains the essential bond between students and staff that has always been the most vital component no matter what changes in governance and organisation have been introduced over the years. These basic principles still apply, just as they have done for centuries. In the words of Pope Nicholas in his Papal Bull founding Glasgow University – words which echo down the ages every Commemoration Day – 'Let a nourishing fountain of learning spring there.'

This should happen, not just in Glasgow, but across the world.

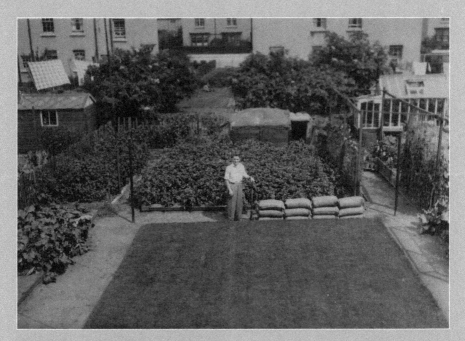

Dad digging for Victory 1940, 62 Thornley Avenue.

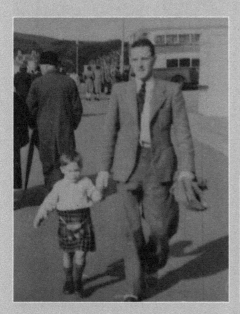

Left: On holiday at Largs with Dad in 1945, aged 4, proudly wearing my first kilt.

Below: Tickets preserved in a family album for the Rangers vs Moscow Dynamos match, 1945 – Moscow Dynamos fielded 12 men, until it was noticed!

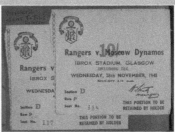

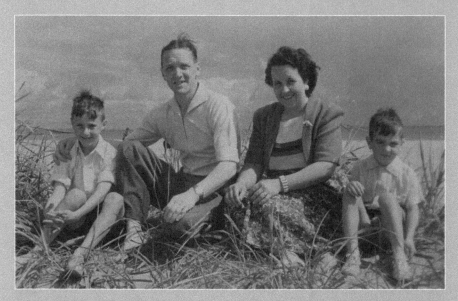

The family on the beach at St Andrews 1950, our last holiday together as a family.

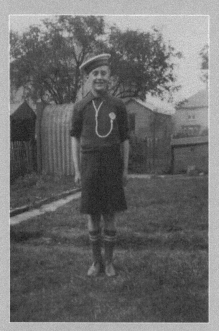

As a life boy aged 13. Note the Anderson shelter behind me, raised from the ground and used as a shed.

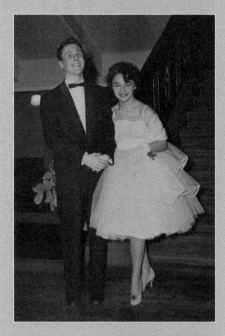

'Daft Friday' in the University Union, 1960. Ann is wearing a dress she created herself.

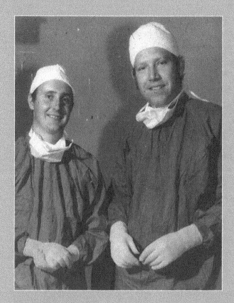

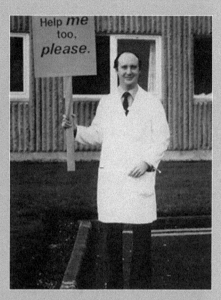

Two surgeons, early 1970s – me standing with (Professor Sir) Peter Bell, who moved to Leicester University a few years later.

Even Professors of Oncology need help sometimes!

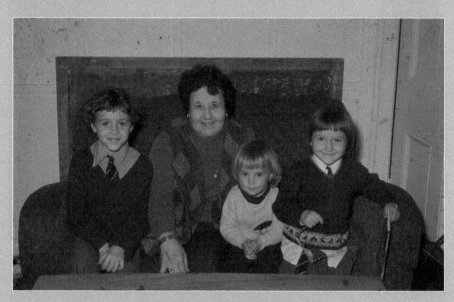

My mother and her three grandchildren, Andrew, Susan and Lynn (L–R), 1977.

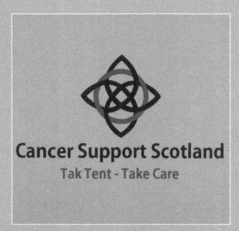

Cancer Support Scotland
Tak Tent - Take Care

The logo for Tak Tent, Take Care Cancer
Support Scotland.

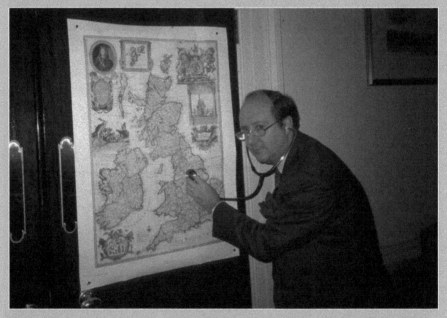

As Chief Medical Officer (CMO) of England, taking the pulse and listening to the state of
health in England.

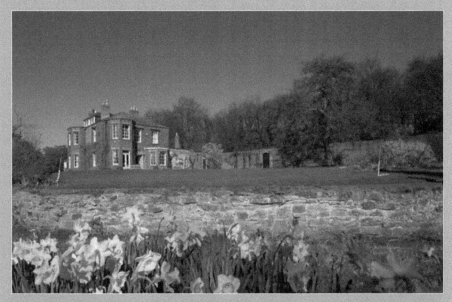

Hollingside House, the Vice Chancellor's Residence in Durham. A previous Canon of the Cathedral, John Baccus Dykes wrote the tune 'Hollingside' here for the hymn 'Jesu Lover of My Soul'.

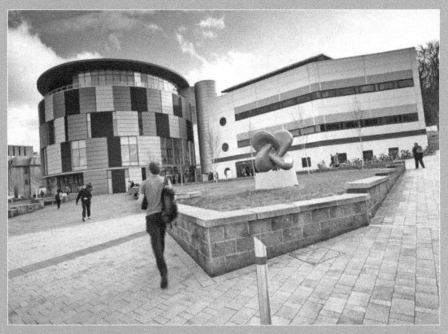

The Calman Learning Centre, University of Durham, opened 2008.

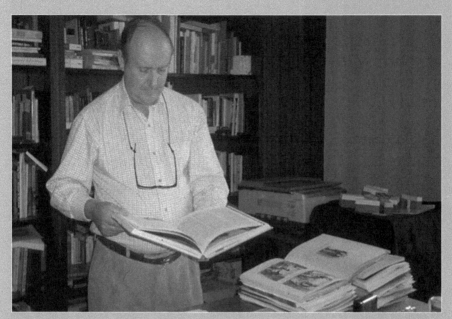

In ny library at Hollingside House.

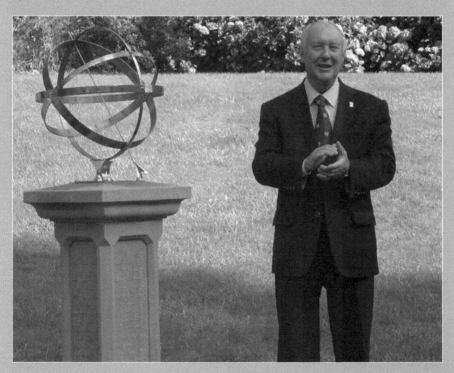

The sundial gifted to me when I stood down as Chair of the National Trust for Scotland; it now sits in the grounds of Brodick Castle on the Island of Arran.

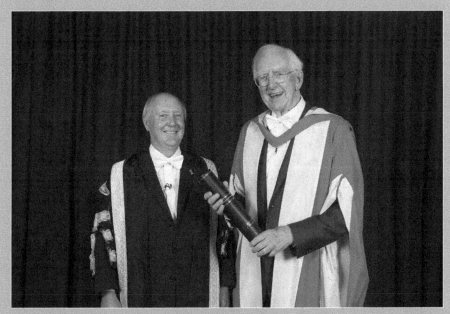

Honorary Graduation of Dr Derek Doyle, pioneer of palliative care, University of Glasgow, 2014.

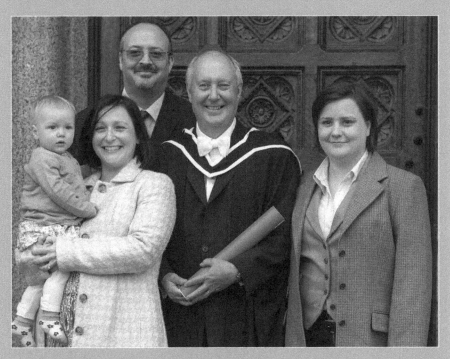

Graduation of Kenneth Calman for the degree of MLitt with his children and one grand-child, June 2013.

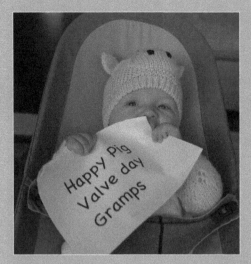

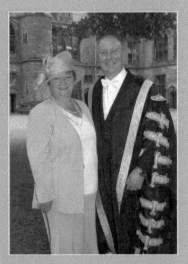

Left: In celebration of the removal of a diseased heart valve in 2007 and replaced by a pig valve. It's happy pig valve day!
Right: Sixty years after we met and still looking young and happy.

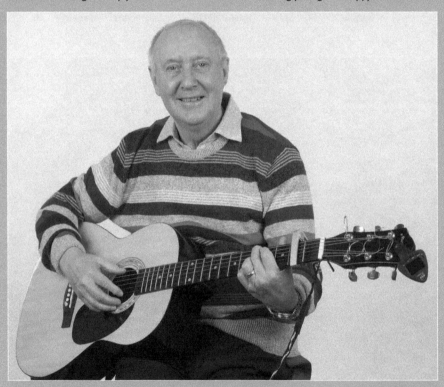

Me and my guitar.

CHAPTER 13

The Arts and Health

THERE IS AN ABORIGINAL proverb which says, 'There are no paths; paths are made by walking.' When I was CMO England, in one of my Captain's Logs, I asked my team what they thought it meant. I can't remember what answers came back, but I have always been clear in my own mind about its meaning. Paths are made by walking just as, for doctors, new forms of treatment are made by discovery, and discoveries can happen in a whole variety of settings: the laboratory, the clinic, the operating theatre, or even in front of the computer.

In my medical career, I have been involved in helping to make three such paths. In all three, I wasn't the one making the initial breakthrough, but was in with the first wave of support, trying to make sure that changes were implemented, spreading the word about them, and helping them to take hold. With the 1970s revolution in medical oncology, for example, I wasn't the discoverer of those life-changing drugs but I was at the leading edge of bringing new treatments to Scotland, where, with Tak Tent, we were the first to establish and demonstrate the value of cancer support groups.

Similarly with palliative medicine: the truly revolutionary work of founding a hospice and spreading the hospice movement was done by people like Dame Cicely Saunders, but both in terms of the care for cancer patients we offered our patients on Ward 7B at Gartnavel, and the palliative care we offered the terminally ill in Victoria Infirmary, we did our best to spread that particular gospel of patient-centred loving-kindness.

And so to the third revolution; the arts and medicine. There is copious literature on this subject, and most of it is about how the arts can be used to improve patients' wellbeing and quality of life. In this chapter, I would like to start off by looking at a different question; whether studying the arts can actually also make someone a better medical practitioner too. That is rather more contentious. Straight away, the question has to be asked; how on earth can you prove it? Conduct a clinical test in which patients' assessments of the empathy levels of a hundred medical students who have read *War and Peace* are measured in randomised controlled trials against the empathy levels of a hundred who have not? Clearly not, and yet I don't doubt that there are huge advantages in medical students taking a short course in the humanities as part of their studies. Please allow me to explain.

I have already briefly mentioned the short course linking Scottish literature and medicine that Professor Robin Downie and I ran for medical students at Glasgow University in 1987.[1] For its time, this really was revolutionary, and from it came the first critical research into the value of the arts and humanities to the training of UK doctors. The original course, which was entirely voluntary, involved a mere four meetings, spread out over several weeks to enable the students to tackle the reading list, which ranged from Seneca's Letters from a Stoic to Robert Pirsig's *Zen and the Art of Motorcycle Maintenance*. Interestingly, although a number of books with medical themes and settings were on the list (for example, AJ Cronin's *The Citadel*, or Chekhov's *Ward 6*), quite a lot of the students thought that this shouldn't be a prerequisite and felt that they benefited from reading material that was beyond their 'comfort zone'. I was delighted by this, as it mirrors a difference I am always keen to point out; the one between training and education. Our medical students could doubtless be trained how to read an ECG, auscultate a chest or put up an IV line, but a true medical education goes beyond that. And literature's ability to take us into minds other than our own, sometimes deflating medical pomposity, sometimes showing the realities of suffering, is a key part of it.

When I became CMO England, I suggested to the General Medical Council that doctors' training should also incorporate a humanities element. In their 1993 Tomorrow's Doctors report on undergraduate medical education, they addressed this by including a special study module on the subject. Robin, meanwhile, was pushing the medical humanities agenda further too. In 1994 he edited *The Healing Arts*, an excellent anthology of poems and prose looking at the many ways in which literature and medicine intersect.[2] Its stated aim – 'to stretch the imagination, deepen the sympathy, and enrich the perceptions of those doctors, nurses, and others who care for patients' – was precisely what we had in mind for the course we had taught together. Not only could literature take medical students inside other people's minds, but it could also show the realities of life in the places they lived – which, given that even today only 6 per cent of doctors come from a working-class background, might well be very different from their own. As Robin and I wrote in *The Lancet*, 'Literature and the arts enable doctors to get outside the professional cocoon to the harsh world in which patients live.'[3] The shorthand term for using literature or the arts in medical education became 'medical humanities', and in 1997 Robin also co-organised the first conference on the topic held by a Royal College.[4]

As Chief Medical Officer for England, I wanted to push the medical humanities agenda further by taking a closer look at what other practical benefits it could bring. I invited a number of people to a meeting in the Department of Health in Whitehall to discuss this. An 'arts for health' strategy could, I felt, help complement scientific and technological models of diagnosis and treatment. Who knew what benefits could flow from that? Could the arts actually be prescribed, perhaps to reduce patients' dependence on psychotropic medication or to treat depression? Would a short course in literature actually result in more compassionate and intuitive doctors – or was that wishful thinking? I wanted to find out.

In March 1998, with the help of the John Wyn Owen and the Nuffield Trust, we held a conference on 'The Humanities in Medicine' at Windsor. Its purpose was threefold: to look at the role of the arts in medical student education, individual health care and community development.[5] There were already, I should emphasise, a number of initiatives along such lines, not least on beautifying old hospitals, funding works of art for new hospitals, and trying to improve the aesthetic appeal of such buildings. Equally, fears had long been expressed – not least by my great hero, Sir William Osler – that a purely scientific medical education wouldn't leave room for students to develop the humanity necessary to do their job properly. The debate about medical humanities, in other words, was already taking place long before the conference assembled.

Yet that conference, attended by a wide range of health profession-als as well as artists, philosophers and theologians, did indeed push things forward. As a result of it, and a follow-up conference the year after, not only was an organisation – the Nuffield Forum for the Med-ical Humanities – set up, embodying its aspirations, but a quarterly journal, Medical Humanities, was also launched. By the time of the second Windsor conference in 1999, I was working as vice-chancellor at Durham, where, as I have already mentioned, we were able to set up a Centre for the Arts and Humanities in the Health and Medicine, which is still going strong. Today there are many such organisations worldwide.

Why does all of this matter so much to me? There are a number of reasons. On a personal level, I have always been interested in the arts, especially literature. Somehow, even when my job as CMO England was at its most stressful, I still made time to read novels as different as Irvine Welsh's *Trainspotting* and Disraeli's *Sybil*. Nor has this love of fiction diminished over the years, if anything, as evidenced by my book *A Doctor's Line*, which looks at seven whole centuries of health and medicine in Scotland through the prism of its literature, it has actually increased.[6]

There has sometimes been, I must admit, a didactic purpose to some of my reading: *A Doctor's Line* began as a commonplace book to guide my thoughts about that 1987 course I taught with Robin. But over the years I have become even more convinced about its central message, which is one I spell out in the book's concluding chapter:

As medicine becomes more and more technical, science-based and evidence-driven, there remains a need to assert its humanity, and the importance of caring and compassion. For many young doctors this will be through the example of their seniors and teachers; role models are critical. But with more and more frequent rotations and changing specialities, and increasing specialisation, it may be more difficult to have an effective mentorship/apprenticeship process. The use of literature... can provide a way of raising difficult issues, allowing discussion and the challenging of assumptions and behaviours.[7]

These days, courses, seminars, and discussions on medical humanities occur with increasing frequency, and bright, fact-filled medical students find them a wonderful release, enabling them to think of quality of life and clinical issues in a different way. Such events stimulate their imagination, curiosity and creativity, all things which are central to the role and aim of the doctor.

This kind of melding of CP Snow's 'Two Cultures' was often found in the past, when it was not unusual for doctors to have already taken an arts degree before they started their medical studies, and was implicit in the generalist tradition of Scottish education as described in George Davie's *The Democratic Intellect*. But those pessimists who argue that there is no way back from our overspecialised education should be reminded that today's students often have just as great an appetite for a wider education as previous generations. At Glasgow University, for example, medical students have set up their own arts and humanities society, and lots of them are doing intercalated degrees in other subjects (which now include one in arts and humanities in medicine) in between their main medical degree. When I did this, back in the 1960s, I was one of just four medical students in my whole year to do so; these days, there would be about 70 or 80.

One of the very few papers to try to measure the impact of studying medical humanities was published a few years back in the journal *Medical Education*.[8] Though its authors pointed out the obvious difficulty of providing a categorical analysis, they did suggest that benefits of taking such a course might include an enriched view of life-long learning and professional development. The arts, they concluded, open up the broader social aspects of medical practice to scrutiny and offer new, and distinctive ways of exploring professional knowledge and identity. This squares both with my own experience, and that of seeing young medical students intellectually come alive when engrossed in the arts. In Scotland, when our young medical students finally qualify, they can also take advantage of a book of poetry which is tailor-made for them. Published by the Royal College of General Practitioners and the Scottish Poetry Library to honour the memory of Hawick GP Dr Pat Mawson, *The Tools of the Trade: Poems for New Doctors* was distributed to new medical graduates.[9] A wonderful idea, and a tremendous resource for young doctors just starting out on their careers.

A few years ago, I wrote a book entitled *Storytelling, Humour and Learning in Medicine*.[10] As well as looking at how humorous films, videos, books or cartoons can have beneficial effects on our health, I tried to set out the ways in which stories link patient and doctor. The stories people tell the doctor are critical in understanding the problem, and the way in which the story is told back to the patient is just as important. These stories form the basis of their professional relationship. It struck me – and this is hardly an original thought – that stories might change behaviour if delivered in the correct way. The growth of social media and the way it can rapidly reach people and change their ways of thinking and learning, only underlines this. At this point I conceived the 'contagious theory of behaviour change', which begins with the proposition that stories can change people and that ideas, feelings and attitudes are 'caught, not taught.' I made the case for a contagious agent, the Transmid – the 'transmitted idea' – as the vehicle for change, and that the story, delivered in multiple ways, is the agent itself. Harvard psychologist Howard Gardner's book *Leading Minds: An Anatomy of Leadership* showed how leaders from Margaret Mead to Jean Monnet have used stories to change behaviour, although the best examples of this remain the parables of Jesus or the wide range of children's fables.[11]

The contagion analogy also works if we consider people as Transmids as well as their stories. The most effective ones are often high-profile people who are good communicators. Anne Diamond's campaign against cot death, Cicely Saunders's campaign for hospices are both powerful examples, and so (as we shall see) is Sally Magnusson's Playlist for Life campaign for people with dementia. I have always been much lower profile, but maybe in a small way I have been a Transmid myself, and looking back, I can see quite easily how I was drawn to all three of those medical revolutions I have mentioned. All of them insist that a human being is more than a symptom and should be treated accordingly. Studying medical humanities makes that immediately obvious, while both Tak Tent and palliative care put the patient first in ways which should have been obvious at the time, but weren't.

Turning away from medical education to look at the wider links between the arts and health, it is easy to see how much more important these have become over the last 30 years. Take hospital architecture. Even though it still leaves much to be desired, we are so much better served than we were in the 1970s. Back then, even basic functionality couldn't be taken for granted. When we moved into Ward 7B at Gartnavel, for example, it was a brand-new building, yet some of the doors were too narrow to get all the equipment we needed through and the internal windows between the ward and the corridor were so high up that nursing staff couldn't easily see in. Now, however, functionality is usually in with the bricks, and aesthetics often gets a look-in too. Not only has hospital architecture improved, but within their buildings you can also often find sculpture, paintings and the visual arts, events such as poetry readings, music and even, on occasions, theatre.

From a UK perspective, the most comprehensive recent overview of arts and health is to be found in the 2017 Inquiry Report of the all-party parliamentary group on Arts, Health and Wellbeing.[12] The arts, it claims, have many uses: they can help the elderly stay healthy and independent; enable patients to take a more active role in their own care; improve recovery from illness; enhance mental health; improve social care; mitigate social isolation and loneliness, promote more cohesive communities; enable more cost-effective use of NHS resources; relieve pressure on GP services; while those new and better-designed hospitals can actually enhance the quality of the built environment. That's a long and far from comprehensive list, but its main points are clear. As well as providing a release from pain and sickness, being able to think and create is hugely important in the midst of illness, and the arts can help. In a similar way, public sculpture, dance, theatre and music can all help to create and build the community into something richer and more cohesive.

As an example of how things are moving on, consider that small but growing part of the arts that is available on a doctor's prescription. Back in 1998, we still needed to find out a lot more about how effective arts for health projects were and what they would cost. Now those kinds of facts are becoming more clearly established, and we are seeing both qualitative and quantitative analysis of a whole series of projects. In Gloucestershire, for example, a project with the charity Artlift allows a number of GP practices to be able to prescribe eight two-hour sessions led by artists to patients suffering from depression and mental health problems. Result? GP consultations from the affected group dropped by 37 per cent, hospital admissions by 27 per cent, higher patient wellbeing rates were recorded and so too, even after payment to the charity, were savings of £216 per patient. As a doctor on a similar project observed, provided that patients feel safe and accepted in a non-judgmental environment, 'what emerges is a very natural peer support that we cannot prescribe'. Because of this, every £1 invested in arts on prescription is reckoned to return a social investment of between £4 and £11. 'The conundrum that we have found ourselves pondering,' says the report, 'is why, if there is so much evidence of the efficacy of the arts in health and social care, it is so little appreciated and acted upon.'[13]

Let me give another example that's particularly close to my heart. My mother loved to paint, and when she was admitted to a hospice in the latter days of her life she continued to do so, painting pictures of roses for her grandchildren and myself. She was so pleased to be able to do it as her last act of love; we were delighted to receive the paintings. Mine hangs proudly in our home on Arran, and I am looking at it as I write this. Arts therapy can help patients of all ages, from children on long-stay hospital wards to young people facing what the Mental Health Foundation has called 'the silent plague of loneliness', to dementia-friendly visits to museums and art galleries. In the UK, one measure of the size of the arts and health sector is that it employs 3,600 artists of all types (visual arts, music and drama) who are accredited by the Health and Care Professions Council. While this might sound like a lot, the 2017 Creative Health Inquiry report concludes that in comparison to countries such as Cuba, Australia and Norway, we are lagging behind.

So more than two decades after the Windsor conference, let's have a quick look at the sheer range of arts activities with a health component. In Scotland, Luminate excels in bringing a whole variety of the arts to older people and stages a biennial creative ageing festival. One of its more recent innovations is its move to establish a network of dementia-friendly choirs, which I'm sure will be a great success. All the evidence suggests that not only do choirs induce a greater feeling of wellbeing in their members than in those who sing alone, but it's an even higher level than recorded for participants in team sports.[14] Music, it turns out, is so deeply hardwired into our brains that even when dementia is well advanced, we still recognise and enjoy music that we first loved many years ago. On realising this, Sally Magnusson – whose memoir *Where Memories Go* is a moving account of how she lost her adored mother to Alzheimer's – started the charity Playlist for Life so that family members and carers can make a playlist of music that holds special meaning for someone with dementia.[15] My own playlist has begun.[16] These playlists can not only be enjoyable to compile but bring back happy memories too – and have reduced the need for psychotropic medicine in care homes by 60 per cent.[17] The charity is currently campaigning to ensure that everyone with dementia has access to their own personalised music by the end of 2020. Some of its aims are mirrored in those of another excellent charity, Music for My Mind (www.musicformymind.com), which is working towards clinical trials proving the cost-effectiveness of such using personalised music in this way. At a time when care for people with dementia (1 million in UK alone by 2021) costs more than that of treating cancer, heart disease and stroke combined, any therapies that boost memories and enhance their quality of life – maybe even delaying the disease's onset – is to be profoundly welcomed.[18]

Music isn't the only one of the arts that can be used in the management of dementia. The Moving Image Archive of the National Library of Scotland contains film from all over the country which can also be used to stimulate the memory and encourage engagement in talking about, for example, where people were born and grew up. Garden design can help too – in many facilities for people with dementia there is little or no access to the outdoors, yet gardens can also bring an added measure of tranquillity,[19] while reminiscence projects, painting and even creative writing classes all have been successfully introduced.

Movement and dance provide another opportunity to improve self-confidence and wellbeing. One example of this is Indepen-dance, a Glasgow-based dance company for people with disabilities, and their carers, to enjoy, express and fulfil their potential through dance. Its aim is to enable participation in high-quality arts provision and improve health, quality of life and opportunities for people with disabilities. There are weekly social and therapeutic creative movement and dance classes, and children, young people and adults who have physical and/or learning disabilities are fully included in the creative process of making, performing and being an audience for dance. My daughter Susan also loves dance and in 2017 huge numbers watched her week by week when she appeared in the TV show *Strictly Come Dancing*. If even some of them took up dancing, the health of the population would be hugely improved.

The Big Noise project, run by Sistema Scotland, and drawing on a model established in Venezuela, is a remarkable example of how music can change people's lives for the better. Funded by the Scottish Government, it involves training children from deprived communities – Raploch, near Stirling from 2008, Govanhill Glasgow from 2013 and Torry in Aberdeenshire from 2015 – to play in a symphony orchestra. Through discipline and teamwork, they learn resilience, confidence and pride, and local performances keep the community involved. Currently, 2,000 children are involved in all three projects in Scotland, and evaluation in March 2015 was ultra-positive: along with the expected increase in musicianship, were increases in school attendance, emotional wellbeing, health and social skills.[20]

All of this adds up to a growing body of evidence that the arts can make a difference. More is always going to be needed, and international perspectives can be valuable.[21] But when we measure the benefit the arts can bring, we must always remember the American physician and polymath Oliver Wendell Holmes's warning against excessively narrow definitions – so true and so much a favourite of mine that I hope you'll forgive me using it again:

The longer I live the more I am satisfied of two things. First that the truest lives are those that are cut rose-diamond fashion, with many facets. Secondly that society in one way or another is always trying to grind us down to a single flat surface.

Patients are indeed 'cut rose-diamond fashion, with many facets' and not just flat surfaces, of interest to the doctor because of a single physical disease, and using the arts to promote health is an implicit recognition of this.

I'll end this chapter with a quotation from another poet-physician, this time a Scot writing more than a century before Holmes. Dr John Armstrong (1709–1799), was born in Castleton in the Scottish Borders, graduated in medicine in Edinburgh in 1732, and moved to London. There, in 1744, he wrote a 1,700-line poem 'The Art of Preserving Health' – a remarkable work, which I would love to see rewritten for the 21st century. Dedicated to Hygeia, the goddess of health, it is made up of four books covering the health implications of air, diet, exercise and the passions. Its last verse neatly summarises this chapter's theme:

Music exalts each Joy, allays each Grief
Expels Diseases, softens every Pain
Subdues the rage of Poison and the Plague
And hence the wise of ancient days ador'd
One Power of Physic, Melody, and Song.

CHAPTER 14

Books and Beyond

YEARS AGO, WHEN I was writing a book on medical education,[1] I went to the National Library of Scotland and asked if it had any medical student notes dating back to the mid-19th century. After a short wait, the librarian came back with some papers on which, in neat copperplate handwriting, a student at Edinburgh University had written up the salient points of a lecture on the use of anaesthesia in childbirth. The year was 1852. The lecturer was James Simpson.

I have already mentioned the short story of 'Rab and his friends', a fictional account of an operation watched by Edinburgh medical students, in which a woman was operated on for breast cancer without anaesthesia. When I was a medical student myself, that story – written in 1859 but set in the 1830s – made a deep impression on me. So too did reading that student's notes in the National Library of Scotland. Because this was fact, not fiction. Here was a student who had sat in front of James Simpson, and taken down precisely what the great man – who had discovered the anaesthetic properties of chloroform only five years previously in 1847 – had to say about treating women in labour.

In the lecture, Simpson explained at what stage chloroform could be used ('when the patient commences to complain of much pain') and how it should be administered ('only during a pain and always withdrawn during the intervals'). But it was the third point that interested me the most. 'Always inculcate perfect quietness around the patient,' he told his students, 'particularly when giving chloroform. When you talk to them you often make them excited.' In other words, the patient might be screaming with pain, but doctors must act with gentleness and thoughtfulness. They must be the very model of equanimity. Nearly 40 years before my other great hero, Sir William Osler, penned his essay on equanimity that also influenced me so much, more than a hundred years before I found out what it meant in practice by watching Sir Andrew Kay at work, here was another Scot setting out its importance, spreading the word about science and making a real difference in people's lives. Indeed, when I add that James Simpson, who later became the first person to be knighted for services to medicine, started off studying the arts for a couple of years before he switched to medicine (as I mentioned in the last chapter, this used to be far more common than it is today), you might begin to think that all the key themes of this book are echoed in his life. Come to think of it, they probably are – but that's not my main point.

Instead, what I want to write about here is where I found all of this out: in a library. And not just any library. Because that Victorian medical student's notes were just one of 10 million manuscripts kept, along with 15 million books, pamphlets and journals, and 2 million maps, by the National Library of Scotland. And that institution matters a lot to me because since 2016 I have had the honour of being its chairman. This has been a great joy to me, as have the many other jobs I have had since my so-called retirement, and in this chapter I'd like to explain why.

Like all other libraries, the National Library of Scotland is in a constant process of reinventing itself: by 2025, for example, it has set itself the target of having a third of its collection available online. Given that the size of its collection will have shot up to 86 million (yes million!) items by then, the scale of the initiative is breathtaking. But so too is the potential readership it will be able to reach – 3.5 billion internet users, rather than just the 37,000 registered readers (26,000 of them in Scotland) that it already has.

When I was appointed its chair in 2016, my friend Dr Jeffrey Jay, a distinguished ophthalmologist, wrote to congratulate me. 'It may be the most important of your jobs,' he wrote, 'arguably the one with the most bearing on the viability of our civilisation.' Certainly, the NLS has an absolutely enormous potential to explain Scotland to the world – even just looking at 1,700 films and short clips in the Moving Image Archive would go a long way to doing that, let alone the rest of the library's amazing collection, 27 million (and counting!) physical items. As for explaining the world to Scotland, surely those 42 million e-articles to which the library subscribes could do some of that job too?

There are still far too many people who don't realise how open this collection now is and what marvels it contains. As John Scally, the National Librarian, has pointed out, digitisation means that 'people in Orkney and Shetland will be able to access the same content as people living within a stone's throw of our premises in Edinburgh'. I'll give you just one example of what that means, though I could easily give hundreds. Suppose that someone wants to look at how Kirkwall in Orkney has changed over the last century. On the National Library of Scotland's website, it is the work of just two seconds to call up two neatly overlaying Ordnance Survey maps of the town and its surrounding fields, one from the present and another from 1903. Move a dial on your screen and you can change the transparency of the overlay: to the left, and the world of 1903 comes back into focus, with the Combination Poorhouse on Scapa Road clearly marked and almost isolated in the open countryside to the south of town. Move the dial to the right, towards the present, and the building is no longer marked as a poorhouse and new estates rise up around it in gentle suburban curves where the fields used to be. No longer is it a poorhouse for 50 people with separate dormitories and a fumigating room to disinfect residents' clothes.[2] Instead, it has been renamed and is an attractive-looking residential home. Now that is just one building on just one road in Orkney – and in Scotland's cities, such changes are far more widespread and obvious. When I repeated this exercise with Knightswood in Glasgow, again using comparative maps, the whole enormous council scheme I knew as a child materialised in neat, geometric street grids out of fields and quarries, hospitals disappeared, industries too, supermarkets appeared out of nowhere. Move the transparency dial between past and present on two such maps and you really do feel the brevity of our lives. It is also one of the most immediate and gripping lessons I can imagine in both history and geography, and I recommend that you try it immediately!

I mention Knightswood because that's where my own adventures in reading began – at the library just a hundred yards from our council flat. In 2014, when I published a book, *A Doctor's Line*, which links Scottish Literature and medicine, I returned there to give a talk about it. In hindsight, that was one of the moments when this book began. Occasionally in our lives, we can find ourselves moving that dial between past and present, and maybe something similar happened when I went into the library as a pensioner and thought back to my seven-year-old self. The gap between the two is, after all, my whole life, and that sudden framing seemed to give it a clearer focus. The previous year I had experienced something similar while walking in Kelvingrove Park with my one-year-old granddaughter Grace. As a child, I had often been taken to the art gallery there. Across the road is the Kelvin Hall, where I had seen the circus as a Christmas treat, heard Billy Graham preach and, just over half a century later, had cardiac rehabilitation after a heart valve replacement. I had walked through the park as a medical student on my way to lectures, and taken our dog for walks there in the first years of my marriage. And now, in that same park but this time with Grace (and I should warn you, I am a very devoted grandad) the dial between past and present seemed quite easy to move.

I was still living in Knightswood when I took the Hippocratic Oath, part of which stresses the importance of 'handing on learning'. That, in turn, chimes in neatly with my own beliefs – and fits in perfectly with chairing the board at the National Library of Scotland, where, to be honest, there is such a great team that I don't need to do too much at all. But one thing I do hope to be able to do on the library's behalf is to constantly emphasise that it is firmly committed to its national remit, and should never just be seen as only benefitting Edinburgh. That part of the job became a lot easier in September 2016, when the library took over part of Glasgow's iconic Kelvin Hall as the new home of its Moving Image Archive. Now, for the first time, we could show treasures from the library's collection in Scotland's biggest city.

This made so much sense. On 25 January 2017, for example, we chose the Kelvin Hall as a venue to exhibit the original manuscript on which Burns wrote 'Ae Fond Kiss'; we could only show it for two hours in the afternoon because we needed to restrict the time it was exposed to light. Not only is it Scotland's most famous love song, but Agnes Mclehose, the woman to whom it was dedicated, was a Glaswegian herself. In 'Ae Fond Kiss', Burns was writing to Agnes before she sailed off to attempt a reconciliation with her husband in Jamaica. He penned the letter to her containing the song with, he wrote, just ten minutes before the postman came to collect it, on 27 December 1791; he knew he would never see her again – 'Ae fond kiss, and then we sever; Ae fareweel, and then forever' – and she knew too. Time was against them, just as time was against showing the letter any longer, but for those two hours at Kelvin Hall, the queues to see a 225-year-old document went out of the door. It was wonderful to see the city reconnecting with a fundamental part of its culture, almost as clearly as if someone was working the transparency slide between the past and present on two overlaid maps.

What else can the National Library of Scotland do to show off the nation's literary treasures (as well, of course, as its cartographic, and cinematic ones too?). That's what it is working out right now. Certainly, Kelvin Hall is living up to our expectations, and we would like to be able to stage more pop-up exhibitions like 'Ae Fond Kiss' around the country (and for longer than two hours). But what more can we be doing at the library's base on George IV Bridge in Edinburgh? Here the problem is that, while the Reginald Fairley-designed building is an iconic example of 1930s classical modernism, it would hardly have been commissioned today. It has, of course, firmly established itself as a much-loved Edinburgh landmark; indeed those monumental Hew Lorimer sculptures on its facade mark it out as one of the most austerely beautiful civic buildings of its era. But these days we require different things from a national library; it still must cleave to its main purpose of being the home for the nation's cultural memory, but it has to be functional too. The ground-floor cafe and information area were welcome new additions a few years back, but we would like to investigate whether further modernisation is possible. Ideally, for example, we would like to have more than three unisex toilets on the ground floor and to have a decent-sized lecture theatre at which we could stage events. We are currently looking at whether such plans are feasible given the architectural complexity of the building and its narrow, split-level city centre site. However the plans shape up, I am looking forward to following them through and doing what I can to support the library; this is indeed a job after my own heart.

I knew it would be even before I began. Just as I was about to leave

Durham in 2007, I was appointed to chair of the audit committee of the British Library, and went on to become the deputy chair of the British Library.[3] This didn't take up a huge amount of my time – the audit committee met about four times a year and the full board about six – but I enjoyed the job enormously. One of the main reasons was that before each board meeting, we would be shown a little bit more about the British Library's collection, it was called 'speed dating'. There would be three of four curators in the room, each with some priceless treasure, and we would be able to see it in close-up and, on a one-to-one basis, find out more about it. This also made me realise what a fantastic job being a curator is; in fact, when I do finally grow up, I have decided that is what I would really like to be! Provided they are properly explained – and sometimes even if they are not – seeing iconic books up close can convey a real sense of the past. In 2013, wearing my British Library hat, I was invited to the opening of the Lindisfarne Gospels exhibition at Durham's Palace Green Library, home of the university's special collections. The exhibition, which in-cluded the seventh-century St Cuthbert's Gospel, the oldest surviving book in Europe, was a resounding success, with 100,000 visitors in just three months. It is rare that past and present jobs overlap so neat-ly, much less in an exhibition that also spoke to my Christian faith and bibliophilia – and when you add the extra pleasure of meeting old friends and colleagues again, you can imagine how much I enjoyed the visit.

When it comes to libraries, I'm with Albert Einstein. 'The only thing that you absolutely have to know,' he said, 'is the location of the library.' He's right. They open minds, are a source of new ideas, and provide pleasure, and they do that for all ages. There is no more essential building block in any community, because they are all places where so many of its various groups – book clubs, language learners, LGBT groups, writers, homework clubs, 'Book Bug' groups and many more – can gather. Of course, the presence of so many groups, and the fact that, in a digital age, students learn by talking and sharing ideas, means that there will be less silence and more discussion, and spaces need to be opened up for this to take place. But while libraries are indeed changing, they are just as necessary as ever. Want to find out about local news, local businesses, maybe how to start your own? It's all in a library. Many are also useful in providing health information, and the Macmillan Cancer Support volunteers in libraries are a model others could do well to copy. At a time of financial cutbacks, libraries are vulnerable – especially community ones – but we must never forget the tremendous social good that they do.

The road from Knightswood to the National Library has taken me to a whole variety of libraries en route. I love visiting specialist ones like the Glasgow Women's Library or the Leadhills Miners' Library, and seeing what discoveries I can make on their shelves. There is, for example, a gem of a library at Innerpeffray, in Stirlingshire which, when it was founded in 1680, was the first free lending library in Scotland. When I visited, open in front of me was Adam Ferguson's *Essay on the History of Civil Society*, the very book I had been looking for! Similarly, in the University of North Carolina, I came across a remarkable collection of the writings by, and about, Robert Burns, and had a wonderful afternoon with them. If 2007 was the year that I rekindled by love affair with libraries by joining the British Library, it also marked a sea change in my life. Technically, I had retired. In reality, I was doing far more widely different and wider-ranging jobs than ever. That is what my retirement has been like ever since.

* * *

I have already mentioned the importance of the Boys' Brigade in life. I joined when I was eight, and though I left when I was 17, I kept in touch with the organisation through Ann, who was one of its national training officers. In 2001, I was invited to be president of the Glasgow Battalion, following in the footsteps of Boys' Brigade founder Sir William Alexander Smith, who formed the Glasgow Battalion from the 12 companies in the city in 1885. In 2007, I was invited to become Boys' Brigade national president. To explain why this meant such a lot to me, perhaps I should tell you the story of a Boys' Brigade captain I met recently, who had just come back from a few days' camping with his company by the seaside. Seeing two eight-year-olds in his company rolling around in the sand, he asked them if they'd never seen sand before. 'No,' they both replied. They lived just 30 miles from the seaside but they'd never seen a beach.

The point of the story isn't just about social deprivation, it's about the fact that all these boys and young men were invariably learning something new, developing self-confidence and potential. In my years as Boys' Brigade President, it was great to see them fundraising for charities, tidying up their local environment, taking the King George VI leadership course, volunteering, playing sports, and putting on shows for parents and friends. Listening to them playing in pipe bands brought back memories of my teenage years when my brother and I did the same in our squad at St David's, Knightswood. The officers – all volunteers, of course – were no less impressive in their determination to improve the lives of young people and give them a purpose. I met both the boys and their officers at prize-giving ceremonies. The highest award is the Queen's Badge, which I was interested to note, is now sometimes presented to winners by their parents. The President's award ranks just below that one, and is given for special merit in a particular area or for overcoming a disability or hardship. I presented some of these awards myself and it was invariably moving to realise just how much these boys had had to overcome in their lives.

My time as President coincided with a number of events to celebrate the 125th anniversary of the founding of the Boys' Brigade by Sir William Smith. One of these was at the National Memorial Arboretum in Lichfield where a Boys' Brigade garden was opened on 21 June 2008. Once more we sang 'Will your anchor hold in the storms of life?' but it was difficult to do so without tears as we remembered whole generations of boys and leaders who had served their communities over the years. In the run-up to the actual 125th anniversary on 4 October, there were many other events, including a dinner at the House of Lords in which Sir Alex Ferguson took time off from his managerial duties at Manchester United and spoke about what his years in the Boys Brigade meant to him. On the day itself, Glasgow Cathedral was packed out for a service giving thanks for Sir William Smith's life.

'If I am to be remembered by posterity,' Smith once wrote, 'I should like it to be as the man who taught people to spell Boy with a capital 'B'. The capital letter, I think, stands for potential, for hope – the hope referred to in the verse from Hebrews 6:19 which provides the Boys' Brigade with its motto and symbol, the 'sure and steadfast anchor' of the soul. Smith's greatness was in seeing the potential of young people and, through radical innovations (for the 1880s) like taking groups of boys on camping trips, helping them to realise it.[4] The Boys' Brigade continues to do valuable work improving the lives of young people everywhere, and to have been their President, attending their annual council meetings and keeping informed about what BB companies were doing across the UK and beyond, was both an honour and a privilege.

By 2008, the number of honorary roles I had been given was beginning to pile up. As well as being President of the Boys' Brigade, chancellor of Glasgow University, and chair of the Commission on Scottish Devolution, I was also appointed president of the British Medical Association and chairman of the National Cancer Research Institute (NCRI). I'll mention the last one first, partly because it may be the one people know least about, but partly because it provides a fascinating model for how I think a whole range of charities, research organisations and government departments with the same interests could all work together.

The NCRI has no money to give away for research, but its board represents all of the major cancer research charities, the Medical Research Council, the Economic and Social Research Council, UK-wide government departments of health, research scientists and clinicians, and – most importantly – patients' representatives. Bringing all of these 20 different groups together, as well as the Association for the British Pharmaceutical Industry, it then looks at the £400 million-plus cancer research funding they have between them (or did in 2008: it's more now), and asks hard questions about whether it is being used as effectively as it possibly could be. Here are two examples which occurred during my period (2008-2011) as chairman.[5]

The first relates to cancer prevention. When you added up the amount of research-funding for basic science compared to that for preventative research, we found, basic research wins by quite a margin. After a lot of discussion, we agreed that government health departments and Cancer Research UK should put significant amounts into a new fund to encourage research on cancer prevention. The second example concerned the difference in funding between research into breast cancer and lung cancer, where breast cancer got significantly more. After talking it over, we were able to create new opportunities and funding for more lung cancer research (including from the Roy Castle Lung Cancer Foundation) without diminishing that available for breast cancer research.

The reason I think this is a model others could do well to follow, is that each participating charity keeps its independence, but can interact and collaborate with others on issues of mutual interest. And because the whole aim is to maximise benefits to cancer patients, it makes a great deal of sense to involve them in the organisation too. At one of the institute's annual conferences – these are now the biggest cancer conferences in the UK – I jointly chaired a session with a patient about a new drug development. The patient's questioning of the ways the drug's impact was to be assessed was particularly helpful and brought a sense of realism to the discussion.

As CMO I had tried, through our 1995 report, to end the postcode lottery on cancer provision, so it was particularly gratifying to become involved in work which brought further integration into the ways in which we dealt with cancer. The NCRI has done tremendous work, with a number of major initiatives on topics such as how best to support cancer survivors, further development of the Cancer Research Database, an informatics programme and a national early diagnosis initiative. While I stepped down from chairing it in 2011, back in Scotland, my own cancer charity work continued, and on 2 November 2012 I opened the Cancer Support Scotland's new centre – in many ways the ultimate realisation of our Tak Tent dream. Sir Harry Burns, the CMO Scotland, gave a speech, I said a few words, rang the chapel bell, and the new £1.5 million Calman Cancer Support Centre was declared open. My granddaughter Grace was there to see it, though she was just a baby. One day she'll realise how proud her grandad was that day.

And as it was before her time, I'd better mention another such time and place; 8 July 2008, the Surgeons' Hall, Edinburgh, when I was installed as President of the British Medical Association. The BMA is habitually called 'the doctors' trade union', but it is a lot more than that, and they are just as passionate about the quality of patient care and clinical practice as they are about matters of remuneration. I had been a member since I was a student and – to underline that last point

– had spoken at part conferences on subjects such as raising quality awareness within the NHS and on doctors' core values. Being its president was a very special job – and to give an idea of how special, my predecessor in the role was none other than the Princess Royal. I was installed by an old friend, Professor Parveen Kumar, herself a former BMA President, and gave a speech illustrated using some of my large collection of cartoons. I took as my theme the BMA's motto 'With head, heart and hand', the phrase its founder, Sir Charles Hastings, used when in 1832 he urged the country's doctors to form an association which should 'have as its main objective the diffusion and increase of medical knowledge in every aspect of science and practice'. Although serious enough in its theme, the cartoons made my point that doctors should also be able to laugh at themselves.

The following day the BMA held its Annual Representative Meeting, where its 500 or so delegates discuss policy. This was addressed by Nicola Sturgeon, who was then the Scottish National Party Health Secretary and Deputy First Minister to Alex Salmond. In her speech she rounded on the Conservatives' market-driven reforms in England and pledged that she would prevent private companies from bidding for Scottish GP contracts. All of this went down particularly well with the delegates, who gave her not one but two standing ovations, with accompanying shouts of 'Why don't you come to England?'. 'English doctors hail Scottish vision of the NHS' proclaimed *The Scotsman* on its front page the next morning, while general council chairman Dr Hamish Meldrum pointed out that while devolution in the United Kingdom in general had been portrayed as the three Celtic nations breaking away from England, with the NHS it was the other way around, 'England has broken away from the rest of the UK'.[6]

So began a year which was already heavily political – the commission on devolution I was chairing got going in April – but which now embraced the politics of health too. I attended a full range of BMA meetings, from council to junior staff, tackling issues ranging from NHS reforms to how junior doctors could handle the implementation of the 48-hour limit imposed by the European Working Time Directive. Issues of training, mental health, abortion, GP pensions, professional regulation were all part of an agenda that also, at the time, included the future shape of devolution in Scotland. I also retained an involvement with two new medical bodies, the Academy of Medical Sciences, of which I had been a founder member in 1998, and the Academy of Medical Educators, which came into being under the joint chairmanship of Dame Lesley Southgate and myself in 2006, and who host an annual lecture in my name.

Meanwhile, in Glasgow, apart from my duties as chancellor of Glasgow University and President of the Boys' Brigade, I was also involved in another key project. The Science Centre in Glasgow was set up in 2001. It is an iconic building on the banks of the River Clyde with an associated 127m tower which, when it is working, is the tallest fully-rotating freestanding structure in the world.[7] Take the lift up to the top, and you can see most of the places that have mattered most to me in my life; Knightswood and Anniesland to the north and the university across the river to the north-east, and even though you can't quite see as far as Arran, there's no more spectacular view of the city. The Science Centre is another cause close to my heart – enthusing young minds with the wonders of science, promoting public understanding of science and encouraging people to take up science-based careers. Imaginative programming has helped, with 'Night in the museum' events, along with projects like the mass-handwashing event involving 3,029 children from 36 primary schools that made the Guinness Book of Records, and an active social programme during the 2014 Commonwealth Games. I was chair from 2007–2011, during which time I helped with a lot of organisational issues, before handing over to Sir Jim MacDonald, Principal of the University of Strathclyde, under whose leadership the Science Centre went from strength to strength.

One of the things which grew out of the Glasgow Science Centre was the broader concept of Glasgow as a City of Science, and I chaired the campaign for this from 2009 until 2015. The concept is not new, but we felt that Glasgow's world-class science heritage (Watt, Kelvin, Lister, Bell, Logie Baird et al) should be built on with a visionary and co-ordinated strategy that would not only boost awareness of, and careers in, science but make the west of Scotland a magnet for innovative industries. Before the campaign's launch in 2010, all of the key players in the sector had been approached and preparatory meetings held at the Glasgow City Chambers, and, along with Lord Provost

Bob Winter, I went to Brussels to promote the city's knowledge-based economy.

Over the next few years, science link-ups within the city continued to develop, a comprehensive website was launched to promote science-based events and ventures, the annual action plan became more focused, while at the same time broadening to include art and design, social sciences as well as science, technology, maths, engineering and medicine. I hope that at some stage Glasgow does indeed become a European City of Science. It certainly deserves to.[8]

As you can probably guess by now, I love the Dear Green Place. The honours the city has given me are ones I particularly treasure.[9] Being chosen to be one of Glasgow's Deputy Lieutenants by the Lord Provost meant a lot to me too. In the absence of the Lord Provost,[10] the Deputy Lieutenant is expected to be on hand to welcome visiting dignitaries and introduce them to other people.[11] I had the pleasure of doing that both for Princess Anne (on a visit to Glasgow Caledonian University) and Prince Charles, who on 10 May 2012 paid a visit to BBC Scotland, where he also memorably read the channel's TV weather forecast for the day.

The one royal visit I most remember, however, happened two months after that, when the Queen came to Glasgow. Because the Lord Provost was travelling in the royal cortege, I was asked to welcome her to the Glasgow City Chambers. It was the Queen's Jubilee, and she had just come from a thanksgiving service in Glasgow cathedral. This is where Glasgow University began in 1451, and in a sense it is where the city began too, as a village clustering the wooden church St Mungo built on that site in the seventh century. It is the only complete cathedral in Scotland to survive the Reformation, thanks to its citizens, who prevented its destruction. My wife and I both love the cathedral as well, and we both worship there. So I felt proud that morning, as I waited for cortège to sweep into Glasgow's George Square at noon, that the Queen had seen the building that is at the heart of the city I love, that she'd been inside it and she had worshipped there too.

As I stood outside the City Chambers waiting to greet her, I could sense the crowd's excitement rising. Office workers gathered at the windows all around, and across the road from me a small crowd started waving Union Jacks. Then the first police outrider appeared and the royal car glided up Hanover Street, turned left and drove round George Square. Cheers rang out, flags were waved vigorously, and I found myself looking at a massed bank of raised mobile phones as I went forward to meet the Queen and the Duke of Edinburgh. Maybe in years to come, other people might look at those pictures and wonder who or what was that man welcoming the royals to Glasgow. I'll give them the answer now. He was a Glaswegian, and never prouder to be one.

CHAPTER 15

My Scotland

THERE'S A CARTOON in our Glasgow flat which shows me listening to Scotland. In it, I have a stethoscope connected to my ears and am holding its diaphragm up to a map of Scotland. But that is, in effect, what the Commission for Scottish Devolution that bears my name was doing from 2008–2009; listening to Scotland and seeing whether there was anything that could be done to help the Scottish Parliament 'serve the people of Scotland better, improve the financial accountability of the Scottish Parliament and to continue to secure the position of Scotland within the United Kingdom.' Those words came from the remit set by the Scottish Parliament itself in December 2007. The commission that it voted by a clear majority (76 votes to 46) to set up, would be independent of any political party and would report to both Holyrood and Westminster. The following year marked the tenth anniversary of the passing of the Scotland Act that had brought the parliament itself into being. It was about time for a check-up.

I was appointed to chair the commission in March 2008, and its other 14 members were named the following month. Although I didn't have any direct connection with any political party,[1] two of the commission members were nominated by each of the three main political parties – Labour, Liberal Democrat and Conservatives – who had voted to set it up. Unfortunately, the SNP chose not to become involved.[2] That, I have always thought, was our loss – but it was theirs too. The politicians on the commission were in a clear minority, but had a wealth of experience: from the Lib Dems we had former Deputy First Minister Jim (now Lord) Wallace and party Convener Audrey Finlay, while we had two peers from each of the other two parties, former Lord Advocate Colin (now Lord) Boyd and Lord Elder and from the Conservatives former Scottish Office ministers Lord James Douglas-Hamilton (now Lord Selkirk) and Lord Jamie Lindsay. But add a retired European Court judge (Professor Sir David Edward), the leader of Drumchapel Housing Co-operative (Rani Dhir), a former chair of the Scottish Youth Parliament (John Loughton), the CEO of the Telegraph Media Group (Murdoch MacLennan), the chair of the National Trust for Scotland (Shonaig Macpherson), the director of CBI Scotland (Iain McMillan), Glasgow University's Professor of Islamic Studies (Mona Saddiqi) and UNISON's Scottish Secretary (Matt Smith) and you can see straight off what a talented team I was working with. Though they had widely different perspectives, every one of them was committed to working out what was best for Scotland. It helped that we all got on well too.

For the commission's conclusions to carry weight, we had to be able to show that we had consulted widely, deeply and openly, so that meant staging public meetings from Stornoway to Ayr, Dumfries to Inverness and Glasgow to Dundee, with a trip across the Border to Newcastle to find out what our nearest and dearest neighbours (remember after Durham, I'm a big fan of England's north-east) made of our plans. We wanted to be as transparent as possible and get evidence from as wide a range of sources as we could.

Very few people ever get the chance to find out what it really is like to take the pulse of a country – and to do so not for any narrow party political advantage but because of a genuine interest in whether such a complicated structure as a nation could be made to work in a fairer, more accountable and more effective way. If you're privileged enough to be offered such a role, there's one thing you realise straight off: the sheer complexity of organisational structures in such a modern, inter-connected country as Scotland. And with each one institution or organisation that we examined, we had to ask; is this the best way of doing things? Is it the fairest, for both Scotland and the UK? Can devolution be made to work better, and if so, on what principles?

As I write this, the UK is in the middle of detaching itself from the European Union. If there's one clear lesson about the whole contentious Brexit process, it is that most people probably never realised the enormous complexities involved in trying to achieve what might seem a very simple political aim. The members of our commission learnt that lesson almost a full decade earlier.

We had been given a year to come up with ways of making devolution work better, and had been provided with an excellent secretariat, headed by Jim Gallagher and Paul Kett. We agreed to meet once a month, and the first thing I decided to do was to break down the subject into five different themes, with a task group of between four and seven commission members attached to each. I chaired the group on general principles, while other groups got to grips with how best to fund the Scottish Parliament, its external links with the UK and EU, whether or how to extend its powers, and how to ensure the commission communicated as widely and effectively as possible.

This wasn't a talking shop. We were genuinely open to change and set off with no preconceived ideas. And while we wanted to hear from as many people as possible in person (two former First Ministers and two former Presiding Officers were among a very democratic mix in over 50 public oral evidence sessions) we heard from hundreds more through questionnaires and written submissions. At all times though, we wanted to make sure that our approach was based on evidence, not just on fixed political opinion. So as well as commissioning our own research, we were guided through the complexities of financial accountability by a team of expert economists led by Professor Anthony Muscatelli, with whom I was to work once again when he became the principal and vice-chancellor of Glasgow University in 2009.

Financing a devolved government in a way that was equitable, efficient and acceptable to two different electorates was always going to be difficult. The obvious way to do so would be to devolve more tax powers. Yet how could this happen when Scotland did not even raise enough tax to pay for the public services it currently provided? Even if it wanted to, Scotland couldn't hike its VAT rates because EU rules stipulate that these cannot vary within a member state. Nor could the population-based Barnett formula used to determine Scotland's funding from Westminster be tweaked any further: already there were resentful murmurings in England at Scotland's £1,500 per head spending advantage. Devolving North Sea tax revenues was rejected as it would make the Scottish budget too dependent on a volatile oil price. Some commentators at the time called for full fiscal autonomy, yet when we published our interim report in December 2008, we pointed out that while this would be feasible for an independent country 'it is not consistent with the maintenance of the Union'. And strengthening that Union was, after all, a key part of our remit.

Devolution, all the evidence showed, had been a success. Opinion polls in 2007 placed a devolved Parliament with tax-raising powers ahead of independence by the margin of 55 per cent to 22 per cent.[3] Holyrood was widely reckoned to have increased accountability and accessibility, and its legislation had proved to be generally effective and better scrutinised. Without a Scottish Parliament, we were told, there wouldn't have been a ban on smoking, free personal care, neglected issues such as land reform would not have been tackled, and tram and rail projects might have been overlooked. Distinctive Scottish policies had emerged on matters such as student tuition fees, warrant sales, fisheries, the environment, and many other topics. As former First Minister Jack McConnell pointed out, whereas in the past Scotland had been restricted to a couple of pieces of legislation a year at Westminster, now our Parliament could prove its worth in a whole number of areas.

But what should come next? What needed to be fixed and what could be made to work better? The canvas was blank. Should the Scottish Parliament ordain a separate Scottish summer time? Did it need a second chamber or any changes in the way it passed laws? Should it control laws on firearms or drink driving or would that cause too much confusion? Were any extra powers needed over broadcasting, and if so what? Could we do anything to encourage immigration? Should pensions be devolved too? Should we tear up the Barnett formula – and if we did, what would we replace it with? There was no shortage of questions, yet we were on a tight deadline to provide answers.

By December 2008 we were halfway through our deliberations, and the preliminary report we published then is testimony to just how open our minds were. We were quite clear, for example, that we needed to find out a lot more about matters like revenue and tax raising, broadcasting, firearms policy, drugs legislation, marine planning and we said as much. But we also said that we hadn't got enough of an evidence base to draw conclusions on many other matters too – lotteries, for example, or speed and drink driving limits, tribunals and health and safety. We couldn't be clearer or more transparent; if you thought, for example, that Scotland should have the option of imposing a 20mph speed limit in her towns or an 80mph limit on her motorways, you needed to get in touch and convince us.

Although the details of reform mattered, the bigger picture mattered even more. And no picture was bigger than that concerning the relationships between Holyrood and Westminster, which was examined in all of its aspects from the role of the civil service, the Secretary of State for Scotland, and relations between MPs, MSPs and MEPs. There was also a review of international comparisons to add to our discussions. An important part of this was a consideration of relationships between UK-wide bodies and agencies.

In the end, we were able to produce a unanimous report, Serving Scotland Better, which was published in June 2009. To square that problematic circle of what powers the Scottish Parliament should be given to raise tax, we suggested a model of funding which was 'within the tax system, consistent with economic union, and suited for devolution'. UK income tax rates, we proposed, should be set at a rate 10p lower for the standard rate (ie 10p instead of 20p) and 30p instead of 40p for the higher rate. A 'Scottish income tax' would make up the difference, with the proviso that if the tax rate was raised across one band it would be have to be raised across all of them. Control over stamp duty and land tax could be devolved, as could a landfill tax, air passenger duty and an aggregates levy, and the Scottish Government should be given extra powers to borrow for capital expenditure projects such as building bridges, schools or hospitals. Among other powers to be handed to Holyrood should be running Scottish elections, control over airgun legislation, drink-driving and speed limit laws, and animal health funding. All in all, there were 24 different recommendations set out strengthen devolution, inter-government co-operation, the Scottish Parliament, and financial accountability. These measures were subsequently used as the basis of the 2012 Scotland Act – which, as the UK government's website points out, 'provided the largest transfer of financial powers from Westminster since the creation of the United Kingdom'.[4]

We were always clear that our conclusions would not stay fixed far into the future; though we would defend them as being absolutely right for the present, we also realised that they were only part of devolution's continuing evolution. Lord Smith of Kelvin (another Allan Glen's old boy) chaired a further commission, appointed in the wake of the 'No' vote in the 2014 referendum on Scottish independence, which recommended that the Scottish Parliament be given further powers, not least to set income tax rates and bands at whatever rate it decided. That commission also consulted widely, with 14,000 emails and letters from the public and 250 submissions from organisations, and although all of its members were politicians, that number now included two prominent members of the SNP.

The Scotland of 2014 was, of course, hugely changed by the independence referendum, and it was only right that the course on which it was setting itself reflected those changes. The Smith Commission was right for its time just as our commission was right for ours. It was a tremendous privilege to be given the first opportunity to develop a strategy for devolution, just as it has been gratifying to see so many of our recommendations implemented. On our last evening, the commission members had a small dinner on which we looked back at our year of taking Scotland's pulse. We had worked well together, and our conclusions had been generally well received by the media. I wondered how to commemorate the occasion.

One of my hobbies is paper-making. I have a press in the workshop of my home on Arran and I make sheets of paper, sometimes with flowers pressed into them. I gave them each a sheet, along with a gold star to represent the good work they had done (all unpaid, by the way). I asked everyone to sign everyone else's piece of paper and to draw a picture related to the Commission's work. Some of the drawings will, I feel sure, puzzle posterity altogether.

So it ended, my year of trying to take Scotland's pulse. But when I look back on it, that whole process links up so clearly to lessons I learnt a lot earlier in my clinical training. First of all, we had to diagnose what was wrong, all the time keeping an open mind and checking all the other symptoms we could discern, constantly communicating with the patient as openly as possible. The first commission's report in December 2008 was, if you like, a provisional diagnosis; nothing had yet been firmly decided; we were having yet more meetings and more information was pouring in all the time. Gradually, though, we started to focus on the key issues, and call on specialist knowledge, just as a clinician might want to do. The analogy isn't perfect, of course. Instead of reading up on the latest cancer treatments, I might find my leisure hours given over to studying the nuances of nuclear energy policy or the complexities of marine dredging, but the workload – the sheer amount of reading involved – was at least comparable. It reminded me of something I once heard said about Sir William Kerr Fraser, my predecessor as chancellor of Glasgow University and a man with a near-legendary ability to master complexity dating at least as far back as his time as Scotland's most senior civil servant: 'A thousand pages in his sight are but an evening gone'. It was almost the same for me. Technically, I was retired, but I was just as busy as ever.

* * *

Just over a year later, I was given another important job in Scotland, and one which introduced me to some places I hadn't seen before. From 2010 to 2015, I was chair of the National Trust for Scotland, and in that time I visited most of its 100–plus major properties, which was one of the great perks of the job.

There is a huge difference between chairing a commission or a committee tasked with sorting out one particular problem relatively quickly – the provision of cancer services in England, say, or the powers needed by the Scottish Parliament – and chairing a long-established organisation. The most obvious is that in the former, all the committee members are starting the task at the same time, and the role of the chair is to bring all the various stakeholders and interested parties together; in the latter, the committee can usually be assumed to have greater expertise. With the Calman Commission, the diagnostic openness I have already referred to came with the proviso that ultimately a fixed point of view had to be agreed. Chairing groups like that, one is always aware of the need to come to a firm conclusion and set a clear strategic course.

In the case of the National Trust for Scotland this had already been done by the review carried out by the Scottish Parliament's former Presiding Officer George Reid, who in August 2010 recommended a radical restructuring of the trust's 'over-governed and under-managed' organisation, replacing its 87-member ruling council with 15-strong board of trustees. As I started my job the following month, my aims were to ensure that this new management structure worked, to support the trust's volunteers, and to do what I could to boost the trust's finances, whether by encouraging more donations or more visits to our properties.

Kate Mavor was an excellent CEO, and had put together a great team, but there was a lot of work to do. For a start, a huge amount of money had to be raised, as only 12 of our 130 major properties were fully funded by bequests. In 2014 we worked out that for the next ten years we would need another £46 million merely to meet our conservation objectives. At a time of austerity, this was hardly easy, and yet we needed to do even more than that. If we were to increase visitor numbers, we also needed to rethink what we could offer them – more play areas for children, for example, more imaginative displays and more engaging guides. We also needed to celebrate those people – 3,000 of them – who worked with the trust as volunteers and made sure that our visitors had the best possible experience. I'll develop the idea more fully later but I have always thought that true, lasting happiness can never be achieved by deliberately seeking it out, but does indeed come from doing something like volunteering. I partly tested my theory when we organised a Happiness Celebration in Edinburgh for our volunteers, when we asked them to come along and write, sing or dance or somehow show and share what made them happy in life. It was a very happy occasion!

The National Trust for Scotland is, I believe, a huge and undervalued asset to the country, and I would love to see it funded as securely as it deserves to be. Although we never had to sell off one of its major properties while I was its chair, there is always a danger that this could happen in the future. Lose part of our heritage, and it's gone forever. Maybe we can get blasé about that. But when you look at what makes tourists come to Scotland, at what drives our biggest national industry, the value of our heritage leaps off the page. Don't ask me how they work it out, but somebody has, and the figure they arrive at to measure what Scotland's historic environment contributes to our economy is £2.3 billion. Yes, billion. That's more than twice as much as agriculture (£758m) and fisheries (£212m) combined.[5] In 2014 I used such figures to call on the Scottish Government to fund a 'national collection' of heritage treasures; I still think it's a good idea.

As well as meeting the trust's volunteers, one of the great joys of being its chair was that I got to see so many of its properties, from the Borders to Unst in the Shetland Isles, and lots of places in between. Some – like the islands of St Kilda and Canna – are magical, with stories to take your breath away. The one question I was invariably asked was which of the properties was my favourite. Knowing full well how deeply people feel about such things, I always managed never to give a direct answer, and I don't think anyone minded, because the NTS really does have such an abundance of great sites. In any case, how do you choose between the wonders of Falkland Palace, the picturesque charm of Culross, the savage beauty of Glencoe or Mar Lodge, the luxury of Culzean Castle, or the closeness to the past that you might pick up at Gladstone's Land in Edinburgh or the Tenement House in Glasgow? The answer is that you can't, or at least not until you have seen them all – which I urge you to do! With my interest in buildings and their history and importance, I was awarded an Honorary Fellowship of the Royal Institute of Architects in Scotland, a very real honour.

But now that I am no longer in the chairman's seat, maybe the NTS's 300,000 members will indulge me if I narrow those choices down to properties which more precisely mirror my own particular interests. And of those, I will pick just four: Burns, gardening, Charles Rennie Mackintosh and Arran. I have always been interested in Robert Burns – indeed, while writing these memoirs I have also been working on a paper looking at his links with Glasgow. So the NTS's Ayrshire properties such as Burns's Birthplace Museum, Souter Johnnie's Cottage, or the Bachelor's Club, where he learnt to dance and debate, are tremendously important to me. Then again, I love gardening, and have done ever since childhood, and the trust has so many superb gardens on its books that it really is invidious to single out any one of them.

We have a small garden at our house in Arran, and from our conservatory, or the man-shed I have at the bottom of the garden, I love to follow the plants keeping track of the seasons. The main NTS property on Arran is of course Brodick Castle, which reopened in 2019 after two years of extensive works, and now has an adventure playpark as well as gardens graced with silver sculptures, as well as, I must add, the sundial that the trust gave me on my retirement. When our grandchildren come up from London, I look forward to watching them enjoy the castle's gardens and playpark, and showing off their grandad's sundial. When we lived in London and were members of the Royal Horticultural Society we visited many wonderful gardens, like Wisley in Surrey and the gardens at Kew, especially at the Christmas Festival with lights and music, and of course in Durham we lived in the Botanic Gardens.[6]

When I visit the trust's properties I often find myself wondering what it would have been like to live in them back in the day. And Brodick Castle, though magnificent, is just too big for me. There is, however, one of the trust's properties that I could imagine living in, and I should explain why. The house I'm talking about is right at the top Upper Colquhoun Street, Helensburgh – G84 9AJ if you want to check it out on Google Maps. You'll see that it's very handy for Helensburgh Upper Station, and there are six trains a day that would take me the centre of Glasgow in about 40 minutes. It's not the busiest railway line in the world but as it is the West Highland Line, it is one of the most scenic. If I want to see Scotland at its best, in other words, catching a north-bound train from Helensburgh Upper would be a great place to start.

If you know anything about Charles Rennie Mackintosh (and as I'm the Honorary President of the Charles Rennie Mackintosh Society, I'm supposed to know a bit), you will realise that Hill House, Helensburgh is the most perfect fusion of his art and architecture. You may recall that my first ambition in life was to be an architect, and how that was fired by going to the same school as Mackintosh. He had trodden a path to influential originality, individuality and meticulous craftsmanship, and my 13-year-old self was hugely influenced by him. Well, some things never leave you, and an appreciation of Mackintosh's style and flair never has (and incidentally, let's not forget that of his artist wife Margaret Macdonald, who created tapestries, antimacassars and gesso panels for the house and whose own genius has until recently been comparatively neglected).

Mackintosh worked on Hill House for two years, from

1902–1904. His client was the publisher Walter Blackie, and, before he drew up the plans, he made sure that it would be entirely suited to Blackie's needs. To work that out, he spent hours following him around in his old house; as well as conforming to the publisher's aesthetic demands for its construction (nothing too predictable, no brick red slate, plaster or wooden beams) the new house would, literally, be purpose-built. Blackie's purposes and mine, while not identical (I wouldn't be as keen on a billiard room), are remarkably similar. As a publisher he needed plenty of shelving for his books, and so would I. I wouldn't necessarily need the huge upstairs flat for the servants, but it wouldn't be too much of a drawback: it's always good to have spare room when the children and grandchildren come to visit. As you can see, I've given the matter a lot of thought.

So does this mean that I'm going to put Hill House ahead of every other property in the National Trust for Scotland portfolio? I'm still not sure. It is just as wonderful as ever, and the steel mesh 'box' that has been placed round it in a £1.5 million conservation process will not only preserve it for future generations but allow visitors to see the building from completely new angles, but it does have one serious NTS competitor. Goatfell. I have climbed up to the granite ridges of the Arran's pyramidal peak a few times now, and I would love to make it to the top one last time, ideally with my grandchildren when they come up from London. It's good to have ambitions, and if I'm spared, this is one of mine.

We'll do it on a clear day, when the sky is a firm, unshiftable blue, yet there's just enough of a gentle breeze to keep the midges at bay. It will be one of those rare days when we'll be able to take our time and not have to rush onwards ahead of gathering clouds, because at my advanced age I'm not going to be rushing anywhere – indeed even walking is going to be every bit as hard as running a marathon was almost half a lifetime ago. We'll take the car from our house as far as we can, then start climbing slowly through the small forest to the thin covering of birchwood and up through the gate in the deer fence and out to rougher, rock-strewn land, with the east shoulder of Goatfell luring us upwards, one step at a time. Then the boulders get bigger and bigger and threading one's way between them becomes harder and steeper, and I'll be beginning to wonder whether it will ever end when all of a sudden the views will open up, and on a clear day like this will be, they will be even more spectacular than ever. Even half-way up, we will have already been able to look back past Brodick and see Holy Island, but now, with any luck, we'll be able to see Ireland itself. 'See that smudge over there on the horizon to the west?' I'll tell the grandchildren. 'That's another country.'

Maybe, when you have imagined a thing many times, you don't actually have to do it. In *Afterthoughts*, my debut poetry collection,[7] there is a poem called 'My Scotland' in which I imagined being on Arran and seeing not only the whole of Scotland, but all of its history too spread out before me. The poem starts in Brodick Bay 'close to where Bruce sailed for Turnberry and then on to Bannockburn'. At Bannockburn itself, on the night of 22 June 2014, exactly seven centuries after the battle itself, Ann and I were there for the opening of the new visitor centre and the Rotunda. The National Trust for Scotland had commissioned Kathleen Jamie to write words that are inscribed on it – 'Come all ye, the country says. / You win me who take me most to heart.' We walked to the Rotunda at midnight, heard the pipes and the prayers, and I couldn't help but think how much my heritage means to me. In my poem, I tried to express this:

> I am a global Scot; at home anywhere
> And, as the story goes,
> 'Where sits the Scot there is the head of the table'
> Free in thought and action
> 'He lives at ease that freely lives'
> In a Nation comfortable with itself
> Confident of its future
> Clear in its vision
> Compassionate and caring, at home and abroad
> An interdependent Nation
> Joined with the world by knowledge, trade, economics
> The environment, health and people
> Scotland a Nation, and in an age
> Beyond independence
> No borders, no boundaries, no barriers
> No limits. So much to do.

My Scotland.
I am now back on Arran, the west side
To finish my story at Blackwaterfoot
With its glorious beach, waves lapping my feet
And the oystercatchers crying,
And the best 12-hole golf course in the world.
Here lies the authentic Bruce's cave,
Where he watched the spider as it tried and tried,
And tried again to reach its goal.
The metaphor is clear.
It is up to us to keep trying
To make Scotland better
With no boundaries, no borders, no barriers,
No limits; still so much to do.
My Scotland.

To get to this side of the island, I might indeed have had to metaphorically climb the one mountain that dominates it; certainly a snow-capped Goatfell is the cover image I chose for the book, and certainly too it would provide the massively wide perspective the poem demands. I wrote it in August 2009, a month before taking up the chairmanship of the National Trust for Scotland, and two months after our Commission on Scottish Devolution published our final report. One way or another, I was thinking a lot about Scotland at the time.

The poem is a full five pages long, which is too much for our purposes here. But it expresses everything I feel about being Scottish: a sense of pride in our past that doesn't tip over into a feeling of superiority; wonder at the sheer natural beauty of the country (the most beautiful in the world, according to a 2017 Rough Guide survey); a celebration of the intellectual curiosity, openness and creativity of its people. In my poem, though, all of this happily coexists with the Union, which gives us the blessing of a wider identity (this was, admittedly, in more optimistic, pre-Brexit days) because 'My Scotland is a broad river flowing to the world'.

The poem doesn't actually specifically state that it is written from the top of Goatfell, but given that it is written from somewhere from which you can imagine seeing Callanish, Solway and the Tweed,

Stirling and Perth, and as the top of Goatfell is the nearest you could ever get to doing this, I'll allow myself a bit of poetic licence. And unless they ask, I don't think I'll explain to my grandchildren just exactly what that is, no more than I will explain precisely what's so special about Scotland, and why it has got nothing to do with shortbread, whisky, and tartan. My guess is that I won't need to. When they – ideally, we – get to the top of Goatfell, they'll see for themselves.

CHAPTER 16

Smile a Lot – It Confuses People

I STARTED WRITING this chapter on a bank holiday weekend at our home on the Island of Arran. The weather had been astonishingly good. For five days, there was sunshine with temperatures up to 23 degrees and not a hint of rain – and all this on the west coast of Scotland too! Ann and I had a glorious walk on Blackwaterfoot beach at low tide with our wee dog Ailsa. What could be better? When we think of happiness, are times like this exactly what we mean? And yet we both knew it wouldn't last, that we would soon have to return to Glasgow and immerse ourselves in the world of emails, meetings, phone calls and work. So was that really happiness?

Happiness – by which I mean deep, fulfilling inner happiness, not just wandering round with a smile on one's face – has always been important to me. My interest in it began many years ago, when I was an oncologist and subsequently as a consultant with an interest in palliative care, and I wrote a number of articles and gave a few talks on happiness, quality of life and well-being. I have also been part of a number of charities which show just how much help can be given to those in need. In the last few years my thoughts have expanded and here I want to explore them more widely. There have been thousands of years of discussion and debate on the nature and achievement of happiness. How could I possibly add anything more? I have found it a difficult, but enjoyable task. One of the key reasons I have been drawn to this subject relates to my love of one of Robert Burns' greatest poems, 'Epistle to Davie':

It's no in titles nor in rank;
It's no in wealth like Lon'on Bank

To purchase peace and rest,
It's no in makin muckle, mair;
It's no in books, it's no in lear, (learning)
To make us truly blest:
If happiness hae not her seat
An centre in the breast,
We may be wise, or rich, or great,
But can never be blest!
Nae treasures nor pleasures
Could make us happy lang;
The heart's ay's the part ay
That makes us right or wrang.

In his fascinating book *The Old Ways*, Robert Macfarlane points out how closely the origin of the word 'learning' draws on a meaning of 'following a path or track'.[1] To learn, then, is to take a path. As you have seen, my life has been full of different paths, many unexpected, and learning has been very much part of this. Learning is the major thing which has made me happiest in life. I don't mean learning in a narrow factual, school-like way but learning about new things, meeting new people, discovering new music, books, art, and ideas – and using that learning. At its simplest, but perhaps most important, learning can also mean watching my children and now my grandchildren growing up. This has provided me with huge amounts of happiness as I have learned to love them more and more. As Burns pointed out, happiness and the heart are very closely related.

That leads me on to another key quotation about happiness, which just happens to come from the Sermon on the Mount: 'For where your treasure is there will your heart be also' (Matt 6:21). Ask yourself where your own treasures are, and your answers will begin to define what happiness means for you and allow you to see if you are spending enough time and energy on each. What is it that is worthwhile for you? What gets you up in the morning? What gives you purpose and meaning? Sometimes, of course, the same things might have a different meaning to each of us. Rabbi Lord Jonathan Sacks tells the story of three men quarrying rocks and when asked what they were doing one replied, 'Breaking rocks.' The second said, 'Earning a living'. The third said, 'Building a cathedral.'

For me, love is a great source of happiness but it takes me to a most difficult topic. What is love? Where does it come from? Here's what Walter Scott has to say about the subject in *The Lay of the Last Minstrel,* Canto Fifth, XIII:

> True love the gift which God has given
> To man alone beneath the heaven:
> It is not Fantasy's hot fire,
> Whose wishes, soon as granted, fly;
> It liveth not in fierce desire
> With dead desire it doth not die;
> It is the secret sympathy,
> The silver link, the silken tie,
> Which heart to heart and mind to mind,
> In body and in soul can bind.

Love is the silver link and the silken tie between us. It has power and energy and that can change things. Giving love to a person, an institution, or a group of people can be challenging, and can require courage, and incur risk. But the purpose is clear: to help and support and be the silver link which brings happiness to others. As a consequence, it may bring you happiness. All of us have the capacity to love and to share the secret sympathy. It is a matter of using that love.

In his great book *A Theory of Moral Sentiments*, Adam Smith shows how being interested in other people, and helping them, can bring happiness to both. Smith develops this theme of the pleasure of mutual sympathy describing 'circles of sympathy': for each of us there will be circles – some big, some small – where our love can help to change things. These circles can be with people, such as families or work colleagues, but they can also include organisations and institutions. The charitable sector has a particular role in this.

Love, it seems to me, is central to happiness, and helping others is an important part of that. Happiness generally involves doing something worthwhile and fulfilling. This can be anything from being in a position of authority in a business enterprise to running a family home or volunteering to do charity work. It implies that your life has a purpose and your values are central to this. John Stuart Mill's autobiography makes the point that 'happy people are those who have their minds fixed on some object other than their own happiness; on the happiness of others, on the improvement of mankind, even some art or pursuit, followed not as a means, but as itself an ideal end. Aiming at something else, they find happiness on the way'. This is exactly what I think too, that happiness is an accidental byproduct of a targeted aim. To the great philanthropist Andrew Carnegie, more important than making a great deal of money – which he of course did – was what you did with it. In *The Gospel of Wealth*, his answer was clear: give it away to good causes. Libraries in Scotland and elsewhere have benefited enormously from his generosity and I personally benefited when I was, as a student, awarded two Carnegie Vacation Scholarships. Being a teacher, no matter what the subject, is another example and a huge privilege. To watch young people grow and develop, gain knowledge and skills and begin to practise their subject as part of a profession is an amazing journey to be part of. It is just the same in a primary school, in learning a sport or developing a special interest in music. The happiness for the teacher is very significant.

Humour might bring temporary happiness, and alcohol or drugs might even do the same. My cartoon collection might make you smile. But would this make you happy? Perhaps for a short while, but all too soon it would be back to the grindstone. Clinical and biological aspects of well-being and happiness, however, need further exploration. Is there a possible molecular basis to happiness? Can it be modified by pills, cognitive behavioural therapy or alcohol? The biology and pharmacology of happiness still need to be understood.

You don't sit back and wait for happiness; it requires energy to make things happen, and without energy there is only entropy and disorder. Happiness is thus a consequence of action and energy, by you or by someone else. Personal happiness may not – and perhaps should not – be the primary objective. Helping others, particularly those less fortunate, is a key aspect. The happiness which this brings you is, however, only a secondary issue. It was not being a professor of oncology which brought happiness to me, but the people I met as a consequence of my job and what I was able to do to help people. Some aspects of my work might seem a long way from happiness: it was often difficult and demanding, and my family didn't see me as often as we might have liked. Recently I heard at a Meeting of Columba 1400, an organisation based in Scotland with a particular interest in helping young people, a special phrase: 'Good people are like candles, they burn themselves to give light to others.'

Sadness will always occur: it is how we deal with it that matters. Books can help and there are two which have been of particular importance to me. *Self Help* by Samuel Smiles, that great Victorian bestseller first published in 1853, sets out the ways in which people from poor or deprived backgrounds have risen to positions of great importance in the arts, literature, science and medicine through hard work and resilience. But he also shows how we can triumph through adversity: as he notes in the chapter on George and Robert Stephenson, 'We learn wisdom from failure much more than from success. We often discover what will do, by finding out what will not do, and probably he who never made a mistake, never made a discovery.' *Creative Suffering* by the Genevan doctor, and pioneer of person-centred psychotherapy Paul Tournier has also influenced me greatly and deserves a far wider readership. In it, he looks at people who, like him, were orphaned at an early age, but who rose above this and prospered, and he develops an important concept – that suffering can bring benefits. The 'benefits of illness' may seem a strange phrase, but Tournier explains what it means. 'Events give us joy or pain,' he writes, 'but our growth is determined by our personal response to both, by our inner attitude.' He notes when dealing with illness that there is a double task for the doctor 'to work towards healing, and to help the patient to make, in Pascal's words, good use of his sickness.' He also redefines the role of the doctor: 'the doctor therefore has two tasks: one is pressing immediate: his scientific, technological task. The other is helping his patient to profit from his sickness to the benefit of his personal development.' Benefiting from illness is a difficult concept to discuss with those who are ill, but it does happen. For example, the knowledge that you have a serious and life-threatening illness may change your priorities, and make you see life in a different way.

Unhappiness might have a whole variety of causes: money, job, family, friends, power, health, relationships, where we live and what we do. Should we blame the State or, as Smiles suggested, recognise that what we might want, but cannot achieve, may be up to us to sort out?

Robert Burns responds to sorrow in a particular way:

Contented with little and cantie wi mair
Whene'er I foregather wi sorrow and care
I gie them a skelp, as they're creeping alang
Wi a cog a guid swats and an auld Scots sang.

So how should we deal with unhappiness and disappointment? How can we tap into the source of love? And wouldn't just getting a better job or bigger car make us happier? Helping others, particularly those less fortunate, might well be more effective. Making a difference is part of this and, as I have noted, love is the motivation for helping others. This raises the important concept of the common good or the commonweal, and our obligations to others. In this context I am drawn to the old Jewish saying – 'Many people worry about their own stomachs and the state of other people's souls. The real task is to do the opposite, to worry about other people's stomachs and the state of our own soul'. Hans Christian Andersen reflects these sentiments. 'To be of use to the world,' he argued, 'is the only way to be happy.'

Another important dimension to happiness is freedom – being able to live your life in the way you wish, subject to the laws of the land. The Declaration of Independence of the United States of America states clearly, that inalienable rights include 'life, liberty and the pursuit of happiness'. Note that the right is not to happiness, but its pursuit. Suppression of feelings and beliefs and the inability to speak freely can take happiness away. This poem, written in the 14th century, says it wisely:

Ah! Freedom is a noble thing
 Freedom lets man have liking (pleasure)
 Freedom all solace to man gives
 He lives at ease who freely lives.[2]

Freedom to live, speak, choose, and to act within the law is to live at ease. Thus the political system is key to this, as is the culture in institutions. A study of the Civil Service showed that the individual's position in the structure is very relevant. Research shows, interestingly, that the lower down the organisation you are, the more stressed you become. That's why I sometimes say, 'I don't get stressed myself, but I think I am a carrier.' To Robert Owen, the utopian socialist behind New Lanark, the role of government is to generate greater happiness. Even though this has not yet been taken up as a policy aim by government, our Office of National Statistics does at least publish measures of national wellbeing. The headings include; education and skills, economics, governance, natural environment, individual well-being, our relationships, health, personal finance, where we live, what we do. Another quotation from one of Owen's contemporaries, a Glasgow woman weaver quoted in the Chartist newspaper *Northern Star* in 1838, puts it in a very succinct way: 'Ask them what is the meaning of the word Politics? Is it not the best way to make people happy?' Over the years our environment has changed markedly: one only needs to consider housing to see that. The terrible conditions in which people lived are well recorded in photographs, as is poverty. These issues remain, and still need attention. There is a responsibility on all of us to do our bit to care for, and improve, the environment and our happiness.

A few months ago, in the middle of the night, I developed some serious physical symptoms and was taken to the accident and emergency department in the local hospital. As I sat in my bed worrying, I thought of God and prayed. My faith matters to me, and has provided me with values by which I have tried to live, and yet I have found it hard to write about. Many years ago I was hugely influenced by John Robinson's *Honest to God*, which I bought just after it was published in 1963, and it introduced me to a number of books which have taken me on new paths and made me think differently. Among them, the writings of Richard Holloway have been particularly relevant in helping me to come to my own view on God and faith and links to scientific enquiry.

Robinson attacked not only the notion of there being a God 'up there' (the 'man in the sky' notion patently didn't square with modern science) but invisibly but potently 'out there' too. God, he argued, echoing Paul Tillich, isn't another separate, supernatural being but the ground of all being. Here's Tillich on what that means:

> The name of this infinite and inexhaustible depth and ground of all being is God. That depth is what the word God means. And if that word has not much meaning for you, translate it, and speak of the depths of your lives, the source of your being, of your ultimate concern, of what you take seriously without reservation. Perhaps, in order to do so, you must forget everything traditional you have learned about God, perhaps even the word itself.[3]

This 'ground of all being', says Robinson, is love, and I follow him in concluding that God is in us, and is expressed in the love we have for others. God is the love within you and me. This completely changes the definition of God from 'the supreme being, a power, a force and the object of worship' to the depth of our own being, associated with love. We must never make the mistake, however, of thinking Man is God – but the love within us is fundamental.

As discussed earlier, everyone has the capacity to love. Everyone can express feelings, feel concerned, want to help others, and help to achieve the greatest happiness for the greatest number. This is the great power of love, which is regardless of race, religion, gender or colour. But it does require action, energy, passion and in some cases personal hardship and sacrifice. Tackling poverty, neglect, prejudice, or racial tension is not easy. Sometimes it requires special skills, but everyone can, and must, be involved if the world is to be a better place.

To me, these aren't just abstract ideas. That night I spent in A&E, I knew that I was surrounded by love. My wife and daughter were with me, and I was being cared for by the hospital's medical and nursing staff, as well as the ambulance team, and all of them had or were showing love to me. Shared love has a particular power. It can be a remarkable resource for change and the promotion of goodwill; a source of energy, passion and power. We can tap into this power through prayer, creating a kind of spiritual internet, connecting people and ideas. This is at the heart of many charities.

How do we learn about love? By accident of birth you may have been brought up in a particular faith background, or perhaps none. In terms of our ability to love, that doesn't matter. As Adam Smith wrote in *The Theory of Moral Sentiments*, 'Howsoever selfish man may be supposed there are evidently some principles in his nature which interest him in the fortunes of others, though he derives nothing from it but the pleasure of seeing it.'

One of the most powerful books I have read is by *The Greatest Thing in the World* by Henry Drummond (1851–1897). When it was published in 1890, it became a bestseller. The greatest thing in the world, in case you're wondering, is love, and the greatest description of love is the one St Paul wrote in 1 Corinthians 13. Drummond covers the characteristics of love expressed by Paul. These include patience, kindness, generosity, humility, courtesy, unselfishness, good temper, guilelessness, and sincerity. The key is to practise these attributes amongst people and to assist with their needs. Drummond recognises that some knowledge will vanish and new knowledge will be discovered. Money, fortune and fame won't last. But love will.

Where does all of this leave churches and organised religion? Are they doomed to become empty, abandoned as terminally boring by their former congregations? There must be a case for denominations of the same faith working together, and indeed links between different faiths. If the primary function of faith is, through love, to improve the lives of all people, then such links matter. They could be put into practice through organising community support for those in need and there are some remarkable examples of this in practice, over the centuries. All communities need leadership through the role of a priest or minister who understands the community and can develop ways in which those in need are cared for. This is the role of the church: to provide a focus for care and love.

There is thus a real need for different branches of the Christian Church to work more closely together and in recent months there have been strong messages from the Church of Scotland, the Anglican Church and the Roman Catholic Church about just that and celebrating unity in diversity. What a power of love they could make together helping those in need and to work positively for the benefit of all. The former Moderator of the Church of Scotland, the Very Rev Dr John Chalmers, made the headlines when he warned that the church faces 'a drift into irrelevance and obscurity' if it fails to connect with younger generations.[4] He argued that a younger generation communicates in different ways, and religious messages on smartphones 'could help sustain people on their spiritual journey'. 'The real truth today,' he noted, 'is that at the intersection of the church and real people, living on real streets, the rubber is not hitting the road and the traditional patterns of church life... are not going to change that.' Congregations were beginning to change, with many keeping their church premises open every day and making a real difference to their communities, but more needed to be done.

There have been a number of important initiatives in which faith leaders have helped those living in poverty or deprivation. In Glasgow alone there is the inspiring story of George MacLeod,[5] whose Iona Community project was rooted in the grimmer realities of life in Govan, and gave a purpose to the lives of many people. In another project, Geoffrey Shaw[6] led a radical experiment in social gospel ministry in the Gorbals, another deprived area of Glasgow, where Richard Holloway also worked, recording in his excellent autobiography *Leaving Alexandria* that while there he realised that 'God was no longer on his supernatural throne.[7] The place to find him was amongst the dispossessed, among the wretched of the earth.' The Salvation Army, founded in 1865 by William Booth, and many other charities should also be mentioned in this context.

More recently, the work by Norman Drummond with the Columba 1400 leadership academy has given help to younger people from difficult backgrounds and allowed them to develop confidence and faith in themselves. The Men's Shed community project which provides opportunities for men to meet others and do things together is another good example of this, and churches with premises could be part of this type of project.

Andrew (now Lord) Mawson's work similarly deserves celebrating. I first met him in the early 1990s when I was Chief Medical Officer in England. He had been appointed minister of the church in Bromley-by-Bow in London in 1987, and it was anticipated that it would shortly close because of dwindling membership. However, he and his wife Susan, completely changed this. They started a healthy living centre, incorporating a dance and art studio, a workshop, a nursery and lots of other activities, whilst retaining the worship. A remarkable achievement.

These examples are merely the tip of the iceberg and are just ones which have interested me. There are thousands of others, in both religious and charitable community organisations. Bringing them together would show just what can be done and how the church, while retaining its worship and faith, can learn from others and contribute to improving the lives of millions of people.

There is an assumption in this discussion that it is the poor and needy who need attention and are always top of the agenda. However, I have met the occasional doctor who might have benefited from love. Likewise, the lawyer, the teacher, the banker, and many others. Those with power and money may not be as happy as they seem, and they also need care and love.

To conclude, even though I can't believe that God is 'up there' or 'out there', I do believe that there is a power, a spirit which binds us all. Love. It is the depth of our being, it is the love within you and me. There remains a need to bring the various churches and faiths together to demonstrate the power that is available if we really work together.[8]

I began writing this chapter on Arran; I am ending it at a holiday village in Cumbria with my two grandchildren and their parents. My grandson, aged two, has just learned a little song which sums everything up.

You are my sunshine, my only sunshine
You make me happy, when skies are grey
You'll never know dear, how much I love you
Please don't take my sunshine away.

So, am I happy? Where are my riches, my treasures? I am happy and my family and friends are the key element in my own happiness. This is where my own paths to happiness go, and included in that is health to allow me to walk the dog and play with my grandchildren, to enjoy the garden and perhaps play golf. I have been blessed too in having a worthwhile and fulfilling occupation which gives my life a sense of purpose. I also love continuing to learn. Helping others has been at the heart of my life, along with teaching and its great joy of seeing young people do better than I ever could.

On top of that, I also have plenty of hobbies on which to focus my energy and expand my interests; currently Scottish Literature, paper-making, sundials and writing poetry. It is important to have time to be quiet and reflect; the most difficult one I use dog-walking for this. Sadness will not go away, it will still occur, and so will anger and disappointment. I have had to learn to deal with all of them.

In Bertrand Russell's words, 'Success is getting what you want, happiness is wanting what you get.' And in my own words, smile a lot – it confuses people and happiness will find you. A poem that I've just come across puts it even better:

Smiling is infectious
You catch it like the flu
When someone smiled at me today
I started smiling too
I walked around the corner
And someone saw me grin
When he smiled I realised
I had passed it on to him
I thought about the smile
And then realised its worth
A single smile like mine
Could travel round the earth
So if you feel a smile begin
Don't leave it undetected
Start an epidemic
and get the world infected.[9]

CHAPTER 17

Cum Scientia Succurro

'There are two important days in your life, the day you are born, and the day you discover why' – Mark Twain

THROUGHOUT THIS BOOK I have set out some of the issues and events which have shaped me, mentioned some of the people who have most influenced me, tried to understand some of my characteristics and values, and why I have been happy. However, I deliberately have not discussed whether or not I feel I have had a purpose in life. I'll try to do that here. I have had lots of opportunities presented to me, often with associated risks, and I have taken them. These wee adventures have been the story behind this book, and this chapter is an attempt to bring them all together and look at what I have learnt as a result.

So what's my world like now? First, my family. My three children are now all married and have delightful partners. Andrew, my son, is an IT professional and lives close to us in Glasgow. He pops in regularly with his lovely wife Barbara, and checks that I am eating properly, and have clean clothes on. Lynn lives in London with her husband Craig. She is a nurse with a PhD, and now an academic with an interest in cancer care and survivorship. I am very proud of her. Craig is special in the Calman family. He is 6ft 2in, about a foot taller than the rest of us, which means that he is very useful at lifting things from high shelves. They are the parents of my two wonderful grandchildren, Grace and Brodie. What a joy, and how exhausting they have been. Susan, my youngest, began life as a lawyer, but gave that up to be a stand-up comedian. She has done rather well and especially after her appearance on Strictly Come Dancing, I am now mainly known for being her father. Lee, her wife, is a remarkably tolerant person to live with her! They get on so well, and it's always wonderful to visit them.

My two grandchildren live in London so it is not possible to see them as often as we would like. We converse on the screen. To see them grow up is fantastic, and though they speak with an East End of London accent, Grace has been having lessons in Glaswegian and can now say, in authentic Scots, 'I'm a wee sausage.' Actually, I'm just a bit more of a sausage than she is, and have been since 2007, when I had open heart surgery in which a damaged aortic valve was replaced by one from a pig. The operation went well, and every year on its anniversary I receive a card urging me to have a 'Happy Pig Valve Day'. My daughter Lynn started what I hope will be a long family tradition, but recently Grace seems to have taken it over.

A particular group of staff who have been of special importance to me are my secretaries. They have almost been part of the family. Not enough is said about such very special people, without whom I could not have done as much. I want to pay tribute to them all, from Marion McLeod, my first proper secretary, with whom I still keep in touch 40 years later, right through to Hazel Quinn and Ann Fleck, my secretaries today. Within the civil service I had a very special group in the secretariat, a private secretary, Dr Felicity Harvey (who has gone on to have a most distinguished career), and a number of others in the team, including a diary secretary who sorted out not just my diary but my travel arrangements. What a resource! Judith Sunter in Durham and Nora McLeod in the National Trust for Scotland helped me in so many ways. I am grateful for all they did for me.

One of the most enjoyable things in my life has been working alongside so many remarkable people in so many different organisations. I will mention just two. The National Cancer Research Institute is a complex organisation to run, bringing lots of groups together, yet Jane Cope, its former director, ran it in an exemplary way and was a pleasure to work with. Then there's the British Library, and even though all its chief executives and chairs were excellent, its board secretary, Andrew Stephens, was so outstandingly efficient that I subsequently sent other board secretaries to have a tutorial from him.

So, people do matter. They add to your life and almost always bring happiness. In particular, my wife Ann, has put up with so much as I moved from job to job. She looked after the children, the house and the wider family. In Lord Patten's recent memoir,[1] he also makes the point of how his wife Lavender helped him and sacrificed her life for his. He comments, 'I regularly count my blessings but perhaps do not celebrate them sufficiently often, or with sufficient noise.' I would echo that in relation to Ann, who has been wonderful.

And then there are the pets. Our first dog was Bart, a flatcoat retriever, a wonderful friend to all the family. He was then followed by two bearded collies, Bonnie and Clyde. They were amazing dogs, and had the capacity to become really filthy in any weather or place. My own favourite was our next flatcoat, Mungo, who took me for walks around Durham, during which I learned to write down my thoughts in my little notebook, some of which subsequently became poems. My current dog is a beagle, born on Arran within sight of the Ailsa Craig, so inevitably is called Ailsa. She is beautiful and so good with the grandchildren. But beagles are difficult, walking with them is slow, and they snuffle everywhere they go. I may be out with her for 40 minutes, but we never seem to walk very far. She also eats everything, and we have to keep food locked up. But we love her, and she gets me out. One aspect of having a dog is that one regularly meets, and gets to know, other dog walkers. We are always rather scruffily dressed, with old hats to keep the rain off, and pockets full of black poo-bags, and when we meet, the conversation is always about what the dogs have been doing rather than what their owners have, so our meetings are always enjoyably classless and politics-free. In our block of flats there are a number of dog-owners and we all meet around five o'clock while the dogs play.

But to return my purpose. My life has been complex and exciting with lots of unexpected opportunities in which my real purpose seems to have been to do the best I could in whatever post I occupied. As my jobs always carried with them responsibilities for those needing care, or in the education of those involved in care, that brought with it the greater purpose of helping people in need. In doing so I found great happiness. When I moved to non-patient or public health organisations, there was a broader purpose of changing and improving the health of populations. When I was involved in public institutions, such as the National Trust for Scotland or the National Library of Scotland, my focus was on helping to improve the places, heritage and culture of Scotland, and to help those looking after them, posts which again brought me great happiness.

Some people may be surprised, indeed disappointed, that there are no stories of intrigue, resignations, secret encounters, arguments and other evidence of malfunctioning in this memoir. This is because there were not many, and in any case it is not the way I work; blaming other people and shouting at them can be counterproductive and slow down the process of change. I suspect that I have often been accused of being too soft, too weak and not aggressive enough to get things done, and there may be some truth in this. But I have always tried to achieve things by being pleasant, rather than nasty. This can be difficult but I have noted a quotation from the Book of Proverbs (Chapter 15:1) 'A gentle answer turns away wrath, but a harsh word stirs up anger'. My approach might not always have been quite enough, but I will try to be more assertive in my old age. I had no grand ambition, and there were some things I might have liked to have done, but was not able to do. But, as always, other doors opened, and a different adventure began. My posts in health, in particular, brought me to areas of real need and I enjoyed helping others in these circumstances.

Lionel Blue, the late rabbi, journalist and broadcaster, used to talk about what he called Jewish archery ('Fire an arrow, see where it lands, and then paint a target around it'). When I read that, I immediately realised that this was the story of my life too.[2] I wasn't ambitious in the usual sense of the word, but I did want to do my best (drawing a target) in whatever job I found myself in (wherever the arrow landed). Problem-solving has been at the heart of what I seem to have done, whether it related to the care of a particular patient, defining ways forward in health, or helping plan the future for an organisation or institution. Lord Kelvin's advice is relevant here: 'When you are face to face with a difficulty, you are up against a discovery.' Being curious and learning – making discoveries – have been my paths to happiness.

I often ask young people what they want to do when they grow up. They inevitably mention a profession, or a career in the arts or in business. I usually say to them, 'That's not the answer! The answer is that I don't want to grow up!' I want to continue to discover new things and try different paths and not grow up too quickly. I don't think I am quite grown up yet.

I was never top of the class, though I was usually in the top segment.

But could I have conceived as a medical student that I would become a professor of oncology, or a chief medical officer, or vice-chancellor of a great university? I don't think so. As Dumbledore says in JK Rowling's *The Chamber of Secrets*, 'It is not our abilities which make us what we are, it is our choices.' I'd agree. So what underlay those choices for me? What set my priorities and most defined my character? What qualities mattered most? This section really ought to be written by someone else, as I'm probably a bit biased!

A central part of my life has been in helping others, whether as a Boys' Brigade Officer, a teacher, a clinician, a public health official or the chair of a public body. Bringing happiness to others relates a great deal to my faith and the need to bring love to others, regardless of who they are. This can be difficult, time-consuming and take you away from families and friends, and yet I would not have wanted to miss those times either. They have brought happiness too – not as a primary objective but as an incidental benefit.

Learning has been at the heart of everything I have done, whether it be chairing a commission or writing a thesis on Scottish literature. It has been my main path to happiness, and even while holding down demanding jobs I still made the time to take three Open University courses. I have also enjoyed teaching enormously, and it is a pleasure to continue to pass on my own love of learning – not just about science and medicine, but the arts and humanities too – to others.

People have been very important to me and professional relationships require openness and an ability to communicate to colleagues, the public and patients. It is good to be nice to people, and smile a lot. I have also tried to enjoy each new job, and put my whole energy into it. Part of this is about leadership and building a team. The power of storytelling is obvious and helps in changing the ethos and vision of the team. Engaging people in the process of change is critical, as is the giving of gold stars. The importance of working hard almost goes without saying. Getting up early helps, and most of this book has been written between six o'clock and nine o'clock in the morning. I am a little obsessive and usually catch the train before the train I wanted to catch. I am always looking for new projects to keep myself active.

Some things have not been easy, and taking risks – for example, in starting a new job or a new project – can be difficult. Sadness also occurs in life. I have been able to overcome these episodes by thinking ahead, and using my sadness as a method of improving things. One characteristic I do think I have is equanimity. I don't often get really angry or annoyed. The ability to remain calm and composed is important and I learned this first in the operating theatre. But it is just the same in the public sector, when difficult issues are presented. My motto for this is 'Keep Calman carry on'.

All of these factors are involved in leadership, which requires developing a vision and a strategy to be implemented by staff or volunteers. My leadership style has varied over the years, and in different posts, sometimes actively leading, at other times using the broader skills and expertise of the leadership team. I have learned much about other people in this process, as well as a lot about myself. Alex Ferguson's words are relevant here:

> My job was to make everyone understand that the impossible was possible. That's the difference between leadership and management.[3]

He also notes his father's advice, which I also follow. In the morning, 'Don't put your slippers on... that's why I put my shoes on, just after breakfast.'

I have been fortunate over the years in having dogs as pets and friends. I walk them regularly, often with the family. But in the mornings and evenings, I do this on my own, and have peace and quiet with my wee dog and watch the change of seasons and the growth of plants and flowers. It gives me time to think, and some of the poems I have published stem from such moments. At our home on Arran I have a small wooden garden shed which gives me even more peace and quiet, and time for reflection. It was only when reading Norman Drummond's splendid book *Step Back* (Hodder & Stoughton, 2015) that I realised that this was what I had been doing – stepping back and giving myself time to go over my actions and thoughts, thinking about my purpose and future, and how I could make a difference. I'm glad I found it and it has added greatly to my quiet time with Ailsa, my beagle. I have still much to learn.

So, am I happy? I hope it comes through in this book that I am. I have always enjoyed what I do and when asked 'What was your happiest job?' I usually reply, 'The one I am doing now.' Even in my mid-seventies I still do lots of things I really enjoy. I am the chancellor of a great university, chair of the National Library of Scotland, involved in a wide range of charities, have a wonderful family, friends and two grandchildren. What more could I ask for?

Will I ever stop 'working'? I hope not. I want to continue to write and read and walk the dog. My physical state may hinder some things. For example, at graduation ceremonies I have to climb a short, narrow and circular stair into a pulpit-like structure, from which to confer degrees, and this is getting more difficult. I have read that David Attenborough has said that when he couldn't climb stairs he would stop filming.[4] I have the same reaction to my small stairs. Perhaps I might add one other reason for stopping being chancellor: if when I get to the top of the stairs and don't quite know why I am there, that might be the time to stop!

What ambitions have I still got? I would like to learn Gaelic, not just to be able to speak it, but to use the language to better understand the literature of Scotland. I have tried several 'teach yourself' books but have not been very successful. I would also like to learn to play the piano. When I was a teenager, I had an old piano, and took some lessons but they were never followed through. Perhaps I might do it now. The third task is also musical: I would love to sing in a choir. Again, I did this while at school, but it would be nice to try again. My inability to read music might be my weak point! I would also like to play a round of golf in Augusta, Georgia. On the TV it looks a wonderful course and I would like to see how it matches up with the courses on the Isle of Arran. I have already mentioned how much I would also like to climb Goatfell again, though this may be difficult. I would also like to learn how to tie a real bow tie! Finally, I would like to continue to write more poems and perhaps publish a second edition of my wee poetry book.

One further thought, this time from Shakespeare, in *Julius Caesar* and spoken by Brutus:

There is a tide in the affairs of men,
Which taken at the flood, leads on to fortune.

Omitted, all the voyage of their life,
Is bound in shallows and in miseries.
On such a full sea are we now afloat.
And we must take the current when it serves
Or lose our ventures.

There is a time when opportunities occur, and it leads to fortune. If you don't take it, life may be lived in the shallows. We must go with the tide or lose out. That is what leadership is about. As David Livingstone said, 'I can go anywhere as long as it's forward.'

The poem 'The Road Not Taken' by Robert Frost sums this up:

I shall be telling this with a sigh
Somewhere ages and ages hence:
Two roads diverged in a wood, and I –
I took the one less travelled by,
And that has made all the difference.

I finish with my motto, Cum Scientia Succurro ('Through knowledge I help others'). This has been the guiding path to happiness throughout my adult life. Using knowledge and skill, the world can be made a better place, and this is what I have tried to do.

Acknowledgements

These memoirs were written for my two grandchildren, Grace and Brodie, to tell them a little about their grandfather, or 'Grumps' as I am usually called. My special thanks go to my wife Ann, and my children, Andrew, Lynn and Susan, who have meant everything to me. They have patiently put up with me and my annoying habits over the years – particularly in dealing with my sense of humour.

Although I kept a daily diary over some of the most interesting years in my career, and even though I have albums of photographs of my childhood and some 9.5mm films taken by my father in the 1940s, there were still a few gaps in my memory, I would like to thank those who helped me fill them in, and especially my younger brother, Norman, who recalls my childhood better than I could. It is also a pleasure to acknowledge the people – family, friends and colleagues – who have helped me write this book. I would particularly like to mention Sir William Reid, Professor Robert Allison, and Dr Felicity Harvey, whose memories have supplemented my own. My dogs have also been important in giving me time to think and reflect on our walks together, although any mistakes in the book aren't their fault or anyone else's.

I would also like to thank my colleagues at all the institutions in which I have worked, especially the Glasgow University Photographic Unit, and the many authors who inspired me, some of whom are mentioned here. My secretaries have also been of invaluable support. Without so many heroes and heroines, mentors and friends, I could not have achieved what I have done.

Special thanks go to David Robinson, who helped develop my stories and the paths I have taken. Thanks also to Luath Press for their encouragement to write and share these stories.

I have enjoyed writing this, and I hope you have enjoyed reading it too.

Kenneth Calman
July 2019

Endnotes

Notes Chapter 1

1 See John MacLeod's excellent *River of Fire* (Birlinn, 2011) for a compelling and comprehensive account of the Clydebank Blitz.

2 The Calman connection with shipbuilding goes back to 19th century Dundee, and as the earliest Calman I can find lived in nearby Monifieth in 1597, maybe deep down we are Taysiders. Then again, as the Calmans are part of clan MacMillan and as their motto is *Miseris Succurere Disco* ('I learn to look after the unfortunate') perhaps we are natural medics too.
There are several small hills in Scotland called Calman, at least one stream in Arran called Alt na Calman. There is even a Calman's Wynd in the village of Pittenweem in Fife named after a David Calman, who lived there in the late 18th and early 19th centuries. There is another Calman story which was told to me by the Irish Ambassador to Britain, and which I have confirmed by a visit to Melk Abbey of in Austria. Saint Calaman (St Coloman) left Ireland to visit the Holy Land and got as far as Vienna in 1012, when he was killed by the Magyars and taken to Budapest and hung on a dead tree. Miraculously, the tree started growing again, so Calaman's body was taken to Melk Abbey and buried there and he became the patron saint of Southern Austria. Interestingly, one of the early Kings of Hungary is King Kalman, a not uncommon name in central and eastern Europe. The late *Times* cartoonist Mel Calman, is of Russian/Jewish extraction and I have some of his cartoons at home.

3 Doll, R and Hill AB, 'Smoking and carcinoma of the lung', *BMJ*, 1950, 2, 739.

4 publichealthengland.exposure.co.

5 https://billygrahamlibrary.org/crusade-city-spotlight-1955-all-scotland-crusade/

6 On the other hand, it is important not to get too sentimental about primary school education at the time. Classes often had over 50 pupils, entry was every six months and it was difficult to progress to senior school. All these matters are well covered in Carol Craig's book *The Tears that Made the Clyde* (Argyll Publishers, 2010).

7 You can see it on the Pathé newsreel if you Google the match. It was a significant victory for Scotland as we'd lost all 17 of our previous matches.

Notes Chapter 2

1 As this was 1963, we did this the old-fashioned way, using logarithms and slide rules. The first pocket calculator was three years away from being invented at Texas

Instruments.

2 Cited in Osler: *Inspirations from a Great Physician by* Charles S Bryan (OUP, 1997).

3 In real life the surgeon Henry Osborne Mavor, 1888–1951. Among the other literary luminaries produced by Glasgow University's School of Medicine Tobias Smollett (1721–1771) and AJ Cronin (1896 –1981).

Notes Chapter 3

1 About £45 in today's money.

2 Iain Gillespie, Arthur Roy and Jimmy Elder went on to professorships at Manchester, Belfast and Keele respectively, Mr Kenneth Fraser and Mr Douglas Clark, both distinguished surgeons known for their kindness to patients and staff, remained in Glasgow, and Colin MacKay CBE became President of the Royal College in Glasgow. Their reputations have already outlived the Western, which was demolished in 2017 as part of a £1billion expansion of Glasgow University.

3 Churchill-Livingstone, Edinburgh 1971.

4 *Surgical Aspects of Haemodialysis* by PRF Bell and KC Calman (Churchill Livingstone, 1974).

5 I've used my surgical status on only one other occasion. Returning home from Liverpool

one night, I got on the wrong train. It terminated at Wigan, too late for any onward connection to Glasgow. After I explained to the Wigan stationmaster that I needed to get back to Glasgow because I had important medical work the following morning, he kindly stopped the Glasgow express just for me. After I'd finished my theatre list the following morning I sent him a thank you letter.

6 *Cicely Saunders: A Life and Legacy* by David Clark (Oxford University Press, 2018). David Clark is the founder of the End of Life Studies Group at Glasgow University's campus in Dumfries. I remember Dame Cicely every time I look at a print of a dove which hangs in our home. It was painted by her husband, Marian Bohusz-Szyszko.

7 Cited (pp 15, 45) in the 2012 *Witness Seminar on Palliative Medicine in the uk c.1970–2010* (2013) ISBN 978 0 90223 882 4 and http://www.histmodbiomed.org/sites/default/files/92239.pdf.

Notes Chapter 4

1 Gordon Hamilton Fairley became the UK's first professor medical oncology as recently as 1971.

2 Professor McVie became president of the European Organisation for Treatment and Research into Cancer, Director General of Cancer Research UK and is director of

Cancer Intelligence; Dr Mike Soukop OBE (1947–2016) was director of medical oncology at Glasgow Royal Infirmary. Kenneth Fearon (1960–2016), later professor of surgical oncology at Edinburgh University, and Fiona Gilbert, now Head of Radiology at Cambridge University, were others on the team who went on to great things. In 1980 Dr McVie moved to take up a post in Amsterdam then moved to a series of prestigious European posts. His position was taken by Dr Stanley Kaye, who took over from me as professor of the Department in 1984, and then moved to a number of senior posts in Oncology in the UK including Professor at the Institute of Cancer Research in London and in 2016 was awarded a lifetime achievement award by the National Cancer Research Institute in the UK. I am delighted to have worked with such outstanding individuals.

3 Professor Roland Barnes CBE (1907–1998).

4 *An Introduction to Cancer Medicine* (Macmillan, 1978).

5 Professor Lucien Israel, who died aged 91 in 2017, was one of France's most distinguished oncologists, with extensive expertise in immunology and lung cancer.

6 Professor Paul Carbone (1931–2002) was president of the American Society of Clinical Oncology and the American Association for Cancer Research.

7 For a more complete account, see the Wellcome Trust's 2007 witness seminar I chaired on 'The Discovery, Use and Impact of Platinum Salts as Chemotherapy Agents for Cancer', which is freely available on http://www. histmodbiomed.org/witsem/vol30. html.

8 *Basic Principles of Cancer Chemotherapy* by KC Calman, JF Smyth, and MHN Tattersall (Macmillan Press, 1980).

Notes Chapter 5

1 Confusingly, there are two Professors Alexander Haddows in this story. The one in the last chapter was the head of the Chester Beatty who kickstarted British research into what became cisplatin. The Alexander John Haddow in this chapter is no less remarkable, but was no relation. The best story of his life is the excellent biographical memoir written by PCC Garnham FRS from which I have quoted here. Its veracity has been confirmed to me by Alexander's son David. It is freely available on http://rsbm. royalsocietypublishing.org/content/ roybiogmem/26/225.full.pdf.

2 See, among myriad examples, the NHS Quality Strategy of May 2010 which aimed to establish 'Mutually beneficial partnerships between

patients, their families and those delivering health care services... which respect individual needs and values and which demonstrate compassion, continuity, clear communication and shared decision-making'. https://www.health.org.uk/node/91.

3 On a Hutton-MacConnachy Travelling Fellowship provided by the Royal College of Physicians and Surgeons in Glasgow.

4 *William A Smith of the Boys Brigade*, by FP Gibbon, p51 (Collins, 1934).

5 *Laidlaw* by William McIlvanney (Canongate, 2013) pp 214.

6 On these she was helped by Jan MacDonald, then Professor of Drama and now Dean of Facilities at Glasgow University. There were also important educational programmes for nurses and doctors on cancer care.

Notes Chapter 6

1 Professor Eric Cruikshank did it from 1972 to 1980, Professor Gerald Timbury followed from 1980–1985.

2 The Goodenough Report on Medical Education, (London, HMSO, 1944).

3 'The Pre-Registration House Office Year: A Critical Incident Study', by KC Calman and M Donaldson, *Medical Education*,

1991, 25, 51–59. I have also written a couple of papers on the topic as well as a book, (*Medical Education, Past, Present and Future*, by KC Calman, Churchill Livingstone, 2006).

4 Described in K Calman et al, *Medical Education*, 22, 1988, 265–269.

5 *Healthy Respect: Ethics in Health Care* by K Calman and R Downie (Faber, 1987; OUP, 1994)

6 See, for example, 'Consent, Dissent, Cement' KC Calman and SAM MacLean, Scot Med J, 1984, 29, 209-211.

7 Derek Doyle, *The Platform Ticket*, (The Pentland Press, 1999).

Notes Chapter 7

1 The Nation's Doctor is indeed the title of an excellent and comprehensive history of the role by Sally Sheard and Sir Liam Donaldson (Nuffield Trust, 2006). Sir Liam followed me as CMO England, the 15th person to hold the job since its inception in 1855.

2 The story of public health in Scotland has slightly different roots. The first CMO of the Local Government Board for Scotland was appointed in 1894, though Scotland's first medical officers of health were appointed in 1862 for Glasgow and Edinburgh. Dr Henry (later Sir Henry) Duncan Littlejohn

(1826–1914) took the job that year in Edinburgh following the collapse of a tenement in the Royal Mile in which 35 people died, and held the job for the next 46 years. (After the tenement collapsed, a voice was heard shouting 'Heave awa' lads, I'm no deid yet!' and a boy was rescued – a quote I used for a talk on public health). Sir Henry was also the city's first police surgeon, taught forensic medicine at Edinburgh University, helped to found the city's children's hospital and is thought by some to have been – along with Joseph Bell – one of Arthur Conan Doyle's inspirations for Sherlock Holmes.

3 Within two years, as CMO Scotland, my 1989 annual report highlighted the fact that lung cancer had, for the first time, overtaken breast cancer as a cause of death.

4 This turned out to be a case of under-reporting and the following year it was added to the list of reportable infections.

5 *The Scotsman*, 24 August, 1988. I actually started work as CMO Scotland on 1 January 1989.

6 Sir Christopher France, *The Times*, 22 February, 1989.

7 The formal opening, by Princess Diana, was in October that year.

8 'Monitoring the Spread of HIV and AIDS in Scotland 1983–94'

by D Goldberg, B Davies and H Allardice, *Scottish Medical Journal*, 1996.

9 *The Nation's Doctor*, p. 206.

Notes Chapter 8

1 I am indebted to Alexander McCall Smith for expanding my vocabulary to include this word, which is which I first came across in his book *Friends, Lovers, Chocolate* (Polygon, 2005, p. 57).

2 UK Trial of Early Detection of Breast Cancer Group. 'First results on mortality reduction in the UK trial of early detection of breast cancer', *The Lancet*, ii, 41 1-416 (1988).

3 Banks review of senior health management, June 1994, p. 32.

4 *The Guardian*, 14 October 1991, p. 23.

5 Haddow Memorial Lecture, 28 November 1988. *Journal of the Royal Society of Medicine* Volume 82 August 1989, 455.

6 'Breast self-examination and breast cancer stage at diagnosis' by D Mant, MP Vessey, A Neil, K McPherson, and L Jones, *British Journal of Cancer*, February 1987.

7 Le Geyte, M, Mant, D, Vessey, MP, Jones, L and Yudkin, P, 'Breast self-examination and survival from breast cancer', *British Journal of Cancer*, 66, 917-918 (1992).

8 Mitchell EA, Scragg R, Stewart AW, et al. Results from the first year of the New Zealand cot death study. *NZ Med J.* 1991;104:71–76.

9 'Can the Fall in Avon's sudden infant death rate be explained by changes in sleeping position?' By Peter Fleming, RE Wigfield et al, *BMJ Clinical Research*, March 1992.

10 Though I should mention the book's title: *Healthy Respect* by RS Downie and KC Calman, (Faber, 1987).

Notes Chapter 9

1 See 'BSE and VCJD: Their Biology and Management' under www/open.edu/openlearn.

2 As well as being Cabinet Secretary, at the time he also was head of the Home Civil Service and had been Private Secretary to two Prime Ministers (Margaret Thatcher and John Major), just as he would be to Tony Blair. Having seen his effortless chairing of those ultra-informative meetings at first hand, it was easy to see why he was so highly rated.

3 From 1985–1989 no herds were infected north or west of a line from Edinburgh to Ayr and in the three other affected areas of the country, percentages were less than two per cent; in the worst affected

areas of England, such as Dorset and Kent, the comparable figure was over 4 per cent.

4 Health in Scotland 1991 (HMSO, 1991) pp. 98–99.

5 The 'bovine scrapie' theory was later discredited as evidence emerged that BSE originated in a genetic mutation in cattle, presumably in the 1970s, that was subsequently passed on through contaminated animal feed.

6 Animal & Plant Health Agency, General Statistics, Dec 2018. The actual figures of confirmed BSE cases are as follows: 1992 31,116; 1993 28,536; 1994 20,322; 1995 12,307; 1996 7,076; 1997 3,846; 1998 2,865.

7 Source: NCJDRSU website www.cjd.ed.ac.uk, 2019.

8 See, for example, *Risk Communication and Public Health* edited by P Bennett and K Calman (OUP, 1999), 'Issues of risk', by KC Calman, *British Journal of General Practice*, January 2001, pp 47-51, 'Cancer: science and society and the communication of risk', *BMJ*, 28 September 1996; or 'Risk language and dialects' by Kenneth C Calman and Geoffrey HD Royston, BMJ 11 October 1997 pp 939–943, and Communicating About Risks to Public Health, Department of Health, November 1997.

9 See, for example, the Australian

National Blood Authority
https://www.blood.gov.au/system/
files/documents/companion-22-
pbm-guidelines.pdf.

Notes Chapter 10

1 The Royal Commission on Medical Education 1965–1968 chaired by Lord Todd.

2 According to Edwin Borman, chair of the BMA's Junior Doctors' Committee, the working group's report in April 1993 was 'one of the most important changes to the medical profession since the inception of the NHS', *BMJ*, 15 May 1993.

3 As with all the leading politicians I dealt with, I found that formality helped, and only on my last day did that change. Until then, I was quite happy for them to address me as CMO rather than use my Christian name, just as I would never, while working, call them anything other than 'Minister' or 'Secretary of State'.

4 Interview by Jack Webster, *Glasgow Herald*, 30 December 1991.

5 See Professor RA Howard's article in *Lancet Oncology*, April 2006, 7, 336–346.

6 See 'Cancer line – an experiment in communication', by Kenneth Calman, *Health Education Journal* Vol 42, No 4, 1984

7 Such policies are often seen as symptomatic of the 'nanny state'. My own views on ethical issues implicit in that term are set out in an essay I wrote many years later. In 'Beyond the 'Nanny State': Stewardship and Public Health' (*Public Health*, 2009, 123, 6–10) I concluded that the state's duty to look after health sometimes means guiding or restricting people's choices, as we have done (successfully, although we can still do better) over smoking.

8 Wakefield et al, *The Lancet*, 1998, 637–641.

9 See for example, 'Selfish anti-vaxxers wipe out years of progress' by Janice Turner, *The Times*, 24 February 2018.

Note Chapter 11

1 Hollingside House was a former home of the Victorian clergyman hymn-writer Rev John Bacchus Dykes, who named the music he wrote for 'Jesu lover of my soul' after the house.

Notes Chapter 12

1 Honorary degrees are decided by the University Senate, who wanted to honour Susan for her work as a broadcaster and comedian, and for highlighting mental health issues and LGBT rights.

2 Sir Neil MacCormick (1941–2009) was a distinguished legal philosopher and, from 1999 to 2004 an SNP MEP. In the election, I won 7,551 of the 12,056 votes. The only other elected university post is that of Rector. The post is for three years and all matriculated students can vote. In my time as chancellor there have been four Rectors – Mordechai Vanunu, Charles Kennedy, Edward Snowden, and Aamer Anwar. Charles Kennedy is unusual in that he was elected for a second term because of his popularity with students, a feat only achieved in the past by Benjamin Disraeli.

3 To be completely accurate: 'Argent on a fess Azure between in chief dexter an open book Proper fore-edges and binding Gules and sinister a garb and in base an oak tree eradicated on its top a redbreast Proper and arrow fessways Or.' On my citation, but not on the shield, is the Calman symbol of a dove carrying a thistle in its beak – which apparently signifies that we are part of the Macmillan clan.

4 These days there would probably be more than 200. The number of students attending graduation days averages about 300.

5 The Randolph Hall is next door to, and smaller than, Bute Hall. It is also the place where a dinner is often held for honorary graduates the night before their degrees are conferred on them. These days, graduates in medicine take the Hippocratic oath in public in the Bute Hall, which is, I think a much better way of doing things.

6 To Professor Christian Kay Emeritus Professor of English Literature (Glasgow) and Jean-Luc Marion Professor of Philosophy and Religion, Chicago.

7 I have also presided over degree ceremonies for the Glasgow School of Art, always a very colourful affair. Following the fire there in May 2014, the degree ceremony was a very emotional one, and was attended by firemen who had fought the blaze, who were given special mention. I have also presided at ceremonies in Dumfries where the university has a campus. These are held in a beautiful church, and there is a nice long procession across the grounds to lunch.

Notes Chapter 13

1 *Literature and Medicine: A short course for medical students* by KC Calman, RS Downie, M Duthie and B Sweeney, Medical Education 1988, 22, pp. 265–289.

2 *The Healing Arts: An Oxford Illustrated Anthology* edited by RS Downie (OUP, 1994).

3 'Why arts courses for medical curricula?' By KC Calman and RC Downie, *The Lancet*, June 1996.

4 For the 400th anniversary of the Royal College of Physicians and Surgeons in Glasgow.

5 See *Humanities in Medicine: Beyond the Millennium*, edited by Dr Robin Philipp, Professor Michael Baum, Rev Andrew Mawson and author, Nuffield Trust Series No 10. The Declaration of Windsor, and further details about follow-follow-up work to it can be found on http://www.artshealthresources.org.uk/docs/arts-health-and-wellbeing-from-the-windsor-i-conference-to-a-nuffield-forum-for-the-medical-humanities/

6 *A Doctor's Line* by Kenneth C Calman, (Sandstone Press, 2014).

7 Ibid, p. 305.

8 'A fresh perspective on medical education: the lens of arts' by Lake, J, Jackson, L, and Hardman, C (*Medical Education* 2015, 49, pp. 759–772).

9 *Tools of the Trade: Poems for New Doctors* edited by Lesley Morrison, John Gillies, Ali Newell, and Lilias Fraser (Scottish Poetry Library, 2019).

10 A Study of Storytelling: Humour and Learning in Medicine by Kenneth C Calman (Nuffield Trust, 2000).

11 *Leading Minds: An Anatomy of leadership*, by Howard Gardner (Harper Collins, 1995).

12 Creative Health: The Arts for Health and Wellbeing, July 2017 (www.artshealthandwellbeing.org.uk/appg-inquiry/Publications/Creative_Health_Inquiry_Report_2017_-_Second_Edition.pdf).

13 Ibid, p. 75.

14 A number of papers were presented on this topic at the 2013 Conference of the British Psychological Society's Division Clinical Psychology: see www.bps.org.uk/DCP2013.

15 *Where Memories Go* by Sally Magnusson (Two Roads, 2014).

16 I've already started my own playlist to be used to stimulate my memory when needed. Musically, it's my life in shorthand: Sibelius's Finlandia, Beethoven's Violin Concerto because they were among the first records I ever bought; Bing Crosby's 'I'm Dreaming of a White Christmas' because of my Christmas Day birthday; 'Will You Anchor Hold?' because of the Boys Brigade; 'The Rock Island Line' because of Lonnie Donegan; 'When the Saints Go Marching In' because of the Clyde Valley Stompers; 'Ae Fond Kiss' because of Burns; 'Mull of Kintyre' because I can see it from of Arran; 'The Durham Concerto' because of Durham University; The Star Wars Theme because of Glasgow University graduations; and 'Amazing Grace' because of my love for my family, and 'Farewell

to Stromness' by Sir Peter Maxwell
Davies because of my love of the
Northern Isles.

17 UK Health Secretary Matt
Hancock, on 6 November 2018
at King's Fund health think-tank
about Playlist for Life's involvement
at the Lillyburn care home, north
Glasgow, and the importance of
social prescribing to reduce reliance
on drugs to treat long-term illnesses.
Quoted on
www.playlistforlife.org.uk

18 The 2017 all-party Creative
Health Inquiry report cited above
says (p. 131) that delaying the onset
of Alzheimer's by five years could
result, between 2020 and 2035, in a
£100bn saving for the NHS.

19 See for example *Designing
Outdoor Spaces for People With
Dementia* by Anne Pollock and
Mary Marshall (Hammond Press,
2012).

20 The audit was conducted by
the Glasgow Centre for Population
Health in partnership with Audit
Scotland, Education Scotland and
Glasgow Caledonian University.
Sistema England is currently
working on projects in Lambeth,
Newcastle, Norwich, Liverpool,
Telford and Stoke.

21 For an international
perspective see *The Oxford
Textbook of Creative Arts, Health
and wellbeing: International
Perspectives on Practice* by Stephen

Clift and Paul Camic (OUP, 2016

Notes Chapter 14

1 *Medical Education: Past, Present
and Future*, by Kenneth Calman
(Churchill Livingstone, 2006)

2 That bit came from a report in
the *Orkney Herald* of 12 September
1883 about the opening of the
workhouse. Historical newspaper
archives are also available online at
the NLS site.

3 The Board was a good one, and
got on well under the chairs, Sir
Colin Lucas and Baroness Tessa
Blackstone and the chief executives,
Dame Lynne Brindley and Roly
Keating. It was a great experience
and I was sad when my second
four-year term ended and I left on
31 March 2015.

4 In 2011 I visited the summer
camp of the 1st Glasgow to
celebrate the 125th anniversary
of that first camping trip – to
Auchenlochan Hall, Tighnabruiach,
on 16 July 1886.

5 During my time at the NCRI I was
often glad of my experience working
on the Statistic Commission from
2000–2007. This was a group whose
function was to be independent
of the Office of National Statistics
and to give public assurance of
the accuracy and validity of data.
I chaired the Review of Health
Statistics Project Board which
considered the way in which
health statistics were generated

and used, and learned much about the relationship between statistics and the targets set by public bodies and produced by the Government, and how these are viewed and understood by the public. The commission developed further and is now the UK Statistics Authority.

6 Cancer survivorship is the special research interest of my daughter Lynn, who is a Principal Research Fellow and Deputy Director of the MacMillan Survivorship Research Group at the University of Southampton.

7 BMJ 2008;337:a725.

8 I am also the Honorary President of a Medical Charity, Tenovus, which awards grants to fund research into a wide range of medical initiatives. These are not large grants, but are catalytic, and provide the background for further funding from other organisations. This is a most effective use of their funds.

10 In 2008 the Lord Provost gave me a special award for services to health. I was also honoured three years later to be invited to give the 'Toast to the Lassies' at the city's Burns Supper at which my daughter Susan gave the reply. A memorable night.

11 The Lord Provosts of Glasgow, Edinburgh, Aberdeen, and Dundee are also lord-lieutenants by virtue of their office. All others in the UK are appointed by the Crown.

Notes Chapter 15

1 I have often been asked whether I would have liked to be a politician. I can see that it's a hugely important job and one where you can make a real difference, and I would have liked that. But which party would I have stood for? Over the years I have voted for almost every party and I'd find it difficult to choose just one. Instead, I have preferred to watch from the sidelines and try to influence things in other ways.

2 I did actually meet the SNP's Constitution Minister Mike Russell MSP, for whom I have great respect, for informal talks in May 2009. Earlier, I had pointed out that his party would have no right to criticise the commission if it did not show any interest in it. The SNP did make a submission to the commission on borrowing powers, although it retained its formal position that the commission was hamstrung by its failure to consider the option of independence.

3 Scottish Social Attitudes Survey 1997–2007, quoted in *The Future of Devolution Within the Union: A First Report*, December 2008, p. 25.

4 https://www.gov.uk/government/publications/2010-to-2015-government-policy-scottish-devolution/2010-to-2015-government-policy-scottish-devolution.

5 Figures quoted in NTS magazine for 2014: the actual figures might have changed since, but the proportions probably have not.

6 I have always been interested in the medicinal properties of plants. One of my favourites is bog myrtle, a plant whose oil keeps off the midges. A few months ago I discovered Anne Barker's *Remembered Remedies* (Birlinn, 2011) which is based on reminiscences of people of the Highlands and Islands about using plants for healing. My favourite was the potato, which was carried in the pocket to cure rheumatism. As the potato wizened, it apparently lost its power to keep the twinges away. I must try it someday!

7 *Afterthoughts* by Kenneth C Calman (Kennedy & Boyd, 2017).

Notes Chapter 16

1 *The Old Ways* by Robert Macfarlane (Penguin Books 2012, p 31).

2 From John Barbour's long narrative poem *The Brus*, written in 1375, translated by AAM Duncan.

3 *The Shaking of the Foundations* by Paul Tillich (Pelican, 1962, p 53).

4 Church of Scotland 'must shift from hymns to smartphones or face obscurity', *Daily Telegraph*

26 November 2017, an article previewing 'Signposts of a Living Faith' by the Very Rev John Chalmers, *Life and Work*, December 2017.

5 *George MacLeod* by Ron Ferguson (Collins, 1990).

6 *Geoff: The Life of Geoffrey M Shaw* by Ron Ferguson (Famedram Publishers, 1983).

7 *Leaving Alexandria* by Richard Holloway (Canongate, 2012, page 120).

8 See also *What's the Use of Churches?* by KC Calman, the Marion Fraser Lecture, 2018, The Scottish Churches Trust.

9 Author unknown.

Notes Chapter 17

1 *First Confession: A Sort of Memoir* by Chris Patten (Allen Lane, 2017).

2 John Launer, *BMJ*, 359, p294, 2017.

3 Quoted in *Leadership*, by Alex Ferguson (Hodder & Stoughton, 2015)

4 *The Daily Telegraph*, 3 January 2018.